Evidence-Based Healthcare

Dedication

This book is dedicated to the memory of my mother who taught me, by example, the benefits of optimism and irony.

For Churchill Livingstone

Commissioning Editor: Peter Richardson
Project Editor: Prudence Daniels
Project Controller: Sarah Lowe
Design Direction: Sarah Cape
Page Layout: Kate Walshaw
Index: Elizabeth Pickard
Copy Editor: Holly Regan-Jones

Evidence-Based Healthcare

J.A. Muir Gray

Director of Research and Development,
NHS Executive, Anglia and Oxford Region

MARINA O'MEARA RN
(503) 630. 6129

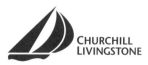

CHURCHILL LIVINGSTONE

NEW YORK EDINBURGH LONDON MADRID
MELBOURNE SAN FRANCISCO TOKYO 1997

A Division of Harcourt Brace and Company Limited.

© Harcourt Brace and Company Limited

First published 1997
  Reprinted 1997 (twice)
  Reprinted 1998

ISBN 0-443-05721-4

British Library Cataloguing in Publication Data
A catalogue record for this book is available from the British Library.

Library of Congress Cataloging in Publication Data
A catalog record for this book is available from the Library of Congress.

Medical knowledge is constantly changing. As new information becomes available, changes in treatment, procedures, equipment and the use of drugs become necessary. The editors/authors/contributors and the publishers have, as far as it is possible, taken care that the information given in this text is accurate and up to date. However, readers are strongly advised to confirm that the information, especially with regard to drug usage, complies with the latest legislation and standards of practice.

The views expressed in this book are those of an individual, and do not represent the views of H.M. Government.

The publisher's policy is to use
paper manufactured from sustainable forests

Printed in the United Kingdom by Bell and Bain Ltd., Glasgow

CONTENTS

HOW TO USE THIS BOOK xi

Finding and appraising evidence

Developing the capacity for evidence-based decision making

Getting research into practice

THE GLOBALISATION OF HEALTHCARE PROBLEMS xiii

Common problems: common solutions

References

CONFESSIONS OF AN AMANUENSIS xv

Reference

ELECTRONIC UPDATES xvii

References

CHAPTER 1 EVIDENCE-BASED HEALTHCARE 1

1.1 The eternal verities: evidence, values and resources 1

1.2 Evidence-based decision making 1

1.3 Evidence-based healthcare – a scientific approach to healthcare management 3

1.4 The growing need for evidence-based healthcare 4

1.5 Barriers to good decision making 7

1.6 Defining the scope of evidence-based healthcare 8
    1.6.1 Evidence-based clinical practice
    1.6.2 Evidence-based policy making, purchasing and management for health services
    1.6.3 'Managed care'

1.7 The limitations of evidence-based healthcare 12

1.8 The limits of healthcare 13

References

CHAPTER 2 'DOING THE RIGHT THINGS RIGHT' 17

2.1 The evolution of evidence-based healthcare 17
    2.1.1 Doing things cheaper
    2.1.2 Doing things better
    2.1.3 Doing things right
    2.1.4 Doing the right things

2.2 The new management agenda: 'doing the right things right' 20
    2.2.1 Strategies that increase the good:harm ratio
    2.2.2 Managing the evolution of clinical practice
    2.2.3 Promoting trials

References

2.3 The impact of science on clinical
practice and healthcare costs   25

Reference

CHAPTER 3
MAKING DECISIONS ABOUT
HEALTH SERVICES   29

3.1 Therapy   29
   3.1.1 Dimensions and definitions
   3.1.2 Searching
   3.1.3 Appraisal
   3.1.3.1 The balance of good and harm
   3.1.3.2 Assessing innovations in health
   service policy and management
   3.1.4 Getting research into practice

Reference

3.2 Tests   34
   3.2.1 Dimensions and definitions
   3.2.1.1 Sensitivity and specificity
   3.2.1.2 Sensitivity and positive
   predictive value
   3.2.1.3 Between a rock and a hard place
   3.2.1.4 Tests: the producer's perspective
   3.2.1.5 Tests: the purchaser's perspective
   3.2.2 Searching
   3.2.3 Appraisal
   3.2.4 Getting research into practice

References

3.3 Screening   46
   3.3.1 Dimensions and definitions
   3.3.1.1 The changing balance of good
   and harm
   3.3.2 Searching
   3.3.3 Appraisal
   3.3.4 Getting research into practice
   3.3.5 Aphoristic warnings

Reference

3.4 Health policy and management
   changes   54
   3.4.1 Dimensions and definitions
   3.4.2 Searching

3.4.3 Appraisal
3.4.4 Getting research into practice

References

CHAPTER 4
SEARCHING FOR EVIDENCE   59

4.1 The searcher's problems   59

References

4.2 The information broker   65

4.3 Coping alone   65
   4.3.1 Becoming a better scanner
   4.3.2 Becoming a better searcher
   4.3.3 Becoming better at critical
   appraisal
   4.3.4 Becoming a better storekeeper
   4.3.5 Use it or lose it

Further reading

CHAPTER 5
APPRAISING THE QUALITY
OF RESEARCH   69

5.1 What is research?   69

References

5.2 Systematic reviews   72
   5.2.1 Dimensions and definitions
   5.2.1.1 Meta-analysis
   5.2.2 Searching
   5.2.3 Appraisal
   5.2.4 Uses and abuses

References

5.3 Randomised controlled trials   78
   5.3.1 Dimensions and definitions
   5.3.1.1 Mega trials
   5.3.1.2 Adaptive design when the
   stakes are high
   5.3.1.3 Patient preference in trials
   5.3.1.4 'N of 1' trials
   5.3.2 Searching

5.3.3 Appraisal
5.3.4 Interpretation and presentation

References

5.4 Case-control studies 87
5.4.1 Dimensions and definitions
5.4.2 Searching
5.4.3 Appraisal
5.4.4 Uses and abuses

References

5.5 Cohort studies 89
5.5.1 Dimensions and definitions
5.5.2 Searching
5.5.3 Appraisal
5.5.4 Uses and abuses

References

5.6 Surveys 93

References

5.7 Decision analysis 94
5.7.1 Dimensions and definitions
5.7.2 Searching
5.7.3 Appraisal
5.7.4 Uses and abuses

References

5.8 Qualitative research 99
5.8.1 Dimensions and definitions
5.8.2 Searching
5.8.3 Appraisal
5.8.4 Uses and abuses

Reference

CHAPTER 6
ASSESSING THE OUTCOMES
FOUND 103

6.1 Five key questions about outcomes 103
6.1.1 How many outcomes were studied?
6.1.2 How large were the effects found?
6.1.2.1 Which yardstick?

6.1.3 With what degree of confidence can the results of the research be applied to the whole population?
6.1.4 Does the intervention do more good than harm?
6.1.5 How relevant are the results to the 'local' population or service?
6.1.6 The clinician's conundrum

References

6.2 Equity 112
6.2.1 Dimensions and definitions
6.2.1.1 Evidence-based cuts at the margin

6.3 Effectiveness 113
6.3.1 Dimensions and definitions
6.3.1.1 Effectiveness and quality
6.3.1.2 Efficacy and effectiveness
6.3.1.3 The patient's perspective: feeling better and feeling happy
6.3.2 Searching
6.3.3 Appraisal
6.3.3.1 Experimental studies of effectiveness
6.3.3.2 Observational studies of effectiveness
6.3.4 Applicability and relevance

References

6.4 Safety 121
6.4.1 Dimensions and definitions
6.4.2 Searching
6.4.3 Appraisal
6.4.4 Applicability and relevance

References

6.5 Patient satisfaction 126
6.5.1 Dimensions and definitions
6.5.1.1 Clinical outcomes: expectations and experience
6.5.1.2 The physical environment: expectations and experience
6.5.1.3 Interpersonal care: expectations and experience
6.5.1.4 Is the measurement of patient satisfaction of any use?

6.5.2 Searching
6.5.3 Appraisal
6.5.4 Applicability and relevance
6.5.5 Evidence-based 'friendliness'

References

6.6 Cost-effectiveness 133
6.6.1 Dimensions and definitions
6.6.1.1 Efficiency and productivity
6.6.1.2 Using outcomes to assess efficiency
6.6.1.3 Marginal and opportunity costs
6.6.1.4 Economic evaluations in research
6.6.2 Searching
6.6.3. Appraisal
6.6.4 Applicability and relevance

References

6.7 Quality 139
6.7.1 Dimensions and definitions
6.7.1.1 Quality assessment by measuring the process of care
6.7.1.2 Quality assessment by measuring the outcome of care
6.7.2 Searching for and appraising evidence on standards of care
6.7.2.1 Searching for papers on quality standards
6.7.2.2 Appraising evidence on quality standards
6.7.3 Searching for and appraising evidence on variations in healthcare outcome
6.7.3.1 Searching for papers on variations in healthcare outcome
6.7.3.2 Appraising evidence on variations in healthcare outcome
6.7.4 Applicability and relevance

References

6.8 Appropriateness 147
6.8.1 Dimensions and definitions
6.8.1.1 It may be appropriate but is it necessary?
6.8.2 Searching

6.8.3 Appraisal
6.8.4 Applicability and relevance

References

**CHAPTER 7
ORGANISATIONAL
DEVELOPMENT FOR
EVIDENCE-BASED
HEALTHCARE** 155

7.1 Key components of an evidence-based organisation 155
7.1.1 The evidence-based organisation
7.1.2 The evidence-based chief executive
7.1.3 Evidence-based everything
7.1.4 Systems that provide evidence
7.1.4.1 The 'evidence centre'
7.1.5 Systems that promote the use of evidence
7.1.5.1 Evidence-based clinical audit
7.1.5.2 Training for evidence-based decision making
7.1.6 Systems that should be more evidence based
7.1.7 Systems for managing innovation
7.1.8 Getting the act together

References

7.2 Evidence-based primary care 167
7.2.1 Improving access: promoting finding
7.2.2 Improving appraisal skills
7.2.3 Building a primary care 'library'

Reference

7.3 Evidence-based purchasing and commissioning 171
7.3.1 Evidence-based needs assessment
7.3.2 Resource reallocation between disease management systems
7.3.3 Resource reallocation within a single disease management system
7.3.4 Managing innovation

7.3.4.1 Promoting innovation
7.3.4.2 Stopping starting
7.3.4.3 Promoting trials
7.3.5 GRiPP – getting research into purchasing and practice
7.3.6 Evidence-based insurance
7.3.7 Black belt decision making

References

7.4 Promoting clinical effectiveness in the NHS 181

7.5 Evidence-based policy making 183
7.5.1 Budgetary pressures – the begetter of evidence
7.5.2 Policies on health service financing and organisation
7.5.2.1 Searching
7.5.2.2 Appraisal
7.5.2.3 Applicability and relevance
7.5.3 Public health policies
7.5.3.1 Does the evidence show an increased risk?
7.5.3.2 Is it possible to reduce the risk?
7.5.3.3 The use of legislation to promote public health

References

7.6 Evidence-based litigation 192

References

CHAPTER 8
DEVELOPING THE EVIDENCE MANAGEMENT SKILLS OF INDIVIDUALS 195

8.1 Searching 195
8.1.1 Competencies
8.1.2 Training
8.1.3 Scanning

8.2 Appraising evidence 196
8.2.1 Competencies
8.2.2 Training

8.3 Storing and retrieving 198
8.3.1 Competencies

8.3.2 Training

8.4 The 'compleat' healthcare manager 199

CHAPTER 9
EVIDENCE-BASED PATIENT CHOICE AND CLINICAL PRACTICE 201

9.1 Clinical decisions as drivers of healthcare 201

Reference

9.2 Types of clinical decisions 202
9.2.1 'Faceless' decision making
9.2.2 Face-to-face decision making

9.3 Evidence-based patient choice 203
9.3.1 The provision of evidence-based information
9.3.1.1 The power of the media
9.3.1.2 Evidence-based information about the process of care
9.3.2 Interpretation
9.3.3 Discussion
9.3.4 Doctors: witch doctors or scientists?

References

9.4 Evidence-based clinical practice 213

References

9.5 Accelerating change in clinical practice 216
9.5.1 Educate to influence
9.5.2 Carrots or sticks?
9.5.3 Growing carrots

References

APPENDIX I
SOURCES OF EVIDENCE 221

A. Published evidence 221
A.1 The Cochrane Library
A.1.1 The Cochrane Database of Systematic Reviews

A.1.2 The York Database of Abstracts of Reviews of Effectiveness
A.1.3 The Cochrane Controlled Trials Register
A.1.4 The Cochrane Review Methodology Database
A.2 NHS CRD Publications
A.2.1 CRD Reports
A.2.2 *Effectiveness Matters*
A.2.3 *Effective Health Care*
A.3 Other good-quality reviews
A.3.1 DEC Reports from the Wessex Institute of Public Health
A.3.2 Systematic reviews from the NHS R&D Programme
A.3.3 Clinical Standards Advisory Group reports
A.3.4 Epidemiologically based needs assessment reviews
A.4 MEDLINE
A.5 EMBASE
A.6 Subject specialist databases
A.6.1 Subject specialist bibliographic databases
A.6.1.1 HealthSTAR
A.6.2 Journals of secondary publication
A.6.2.1 *Evidence-Based Medicine*
A.6.3 Registers of published research

References

Further reading

B. Unpublished evidence: registers of research in progress 233
B.1 The National Research Register
B.2 Database of current health services research

APPENDIX II
SEARCHING 235

Introduction 235

MEDLINE search strategy for asthma/air pollutants systematic reviews 236

MEDLINE search strategy for asthma/air pollutants RCTs 237

APPENDIX III
APPRAISING 239

A. More detailed reading on critical appraisal 239
A.1 Users' Guides to the Medical Literature
A.2 The Cochrane Library
A.3 Standard texts
A.4 *Bandolier*

B. Critical Appraisal Skills Programme – CASP 243

APPENDIX IV
STORING 247

Reference

APPENDIX V
IMPLEMENTING 249

A. Proactive approaches 249
A.1 Main lessons learnt from the GRiPP Project
A.1.1 Choosing the topic
A.1.2 Consulting and involving local professionals
A.1.3 Reviewing the evidence
A.1.4 Acquiring baseline data
A.1.5 Developing evidence-based guidelines
A.1.6 Disseminating and implementing
A.1.7 Evaluation
A.1.8 Project management
A.2 The PACE Programme

B. The reactive approach 254

C. Opportunistic implementation 255
References

D. The rise of 'managed care' 256
References

Further reading

HOW TO USE THIS BOOK

The main aim in writing this book is to help those people who have to make decisions about groups of patients and/or populations base such decisions on a careful appraisal of the best evidence available.

Within the book, a framework has been presented to increase evidence-based decision making within health services. As such, the contents cover three main topics:

1. finding and appraising evidence (Chapters 4–6);
2. developing the capacity of individuals and organisations to use evidence (Chapters 7 and 8);
3. implementation – getting research into practice.

Finding and appraising evidence

In Chapters 4–6, the focus is on the appraisal of evidence about three different dimensions (Fig. 0.1):

- different types of healthcare decision, such as decisions about new treatment services or management changes;
- different types of outcome, such as effectiveness, safety or quality;
- different types of research method, such as systematic reviews, RCTs or cohort studies.

For any problem, all three dimensions must be considered.

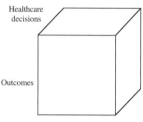

Fig. 0.1

Developing the capacity for evidence-based decision making

In Chapters 7 and 8, ways in which the amount of evidence-based decision making within an organisation can be increased are discussed. This is achieved by developing not only the skills of individuals but also the culture, systems and structures within organisations. These two facets of development are inter-related (see Fig. 0.2).

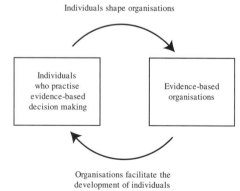

Fig. 0.2

Getting research into practice

Throughout the book there is a focus on implementation, and it is recognised that it is often difficult to implement research evidence within clinical practice and health service management and policy.

The first step is to prepare a healthcare policy (see Fig. 0.3), i.e. a statement of what should happen; for example, that all women aged over 50 years should have a mammogram, or that all people who have had a myocardial infarction should receive a treatment regimen of aspirin and beta-blockers.

Once a healthcare policy has been developed, systems must be designed to ensure that the policy is implemented.

These systems must encompass organisational development and the education of both professionals and the public. The development of systems is always necessary; however, the need to change the culture and structure of an organisation is not invariable.

The preoccupation with productivity and quality that has dominated healthcare management during the last two decades has not necessarily led to the development of evidence-based policies, nor to the implementation of knowledge derived from research for the improvement of the effectiveness, safety, acceptability and cost-effectiveness of healthcare. There is now a general appreciation that decisions made within and about not only health services but also clinical practice must be based on evidence to a much greater degree than they have been in the past such that the knowledge derived from research can be used to improve the public health.

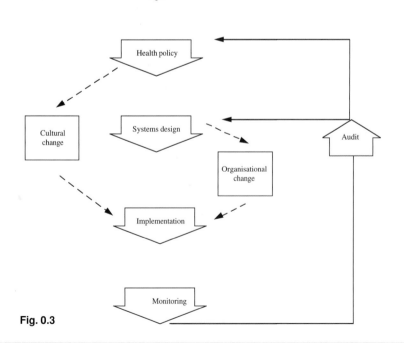

Fig. 0.3

THE GLOBALISATION OF HEALTHCARE PROBLEMS

Although health services appear to differ greatly from one country to another, there are certain common factors that are beginning to influence the evolution of systems of health service organisation and healthcare delivery in all countries irrespective of their geographical latitude.

The challenges to the provision of healthcare, such as population ageing, rising patient expectations and the advent of new technologies, may be obvious in industrialised nations, but these factors also affect Third World nations. A Minister of Health in a Third World country is responsible for providing appropriate services to meet not only the typical health problems of the Third World such as high infant mortality rates, and high mortality and morbidity rates as a result of the prevalence of infectious diseases — problems that were resolved in the 19th century in the industrialised nations — but also the consequences of lifestyle habits such as cigarette smoking, drug abuse and dangerous driving which are predominant in the industrialised societies of the 20th century.

New technologies may be introduced into a Third World country by practitioners or developed in teaching hospitals built in emulation of famous centres in the USA or Europe. These technological developments, however, will be relevant to only a small proportion of the population, although they can consume a large proportion of healthcare resources. Thus, it is vital that health services within the Third World are also managed according to the tenets of evidence-based decision making, although it may prove more difficult to implement such practices and procedures in this situation than within the context of an industrial economy in which private practice, which is much more difficult to influence, is relatively less important than care provided within formal managed systems.

Interventions that have been shown to do more good than harm at reasonable cost but which are not yet widely adopted in countries with developing economies include the administration of aspirin which reduces the health and economic burden resulting from stroke, and vitamin A supplementation which reduces all-cause mortality in children.[1] Conversely, there are other interventions that have not yet been shown to be effective but which are in routine use; these interventions of unproven effectiveness consume resources that could be expended on those which do more good than harm at reasonable cost, such as routine antimalarial chemoprophylaxis during pregnancy.[2] From these examples, it can be seen that evidence-based decision making has a role in the provision of healthcare in all countries, irrespective of the stage of their economic development.

Common problems: common solutions

As the problems associated with the delivery of healthcare worldwide begin to converge, the solutions being sought can be characterised by certain features which are not only evident within the health services of the industrialised nations of the North but also important to the structural reforms of healthcare in the Third World:

- a preoccupation with cost control;
- the development of systems to prevent the burden of cost falling on the individual;
- an increasing authority being given to the function of purchasing healthcare either for people who live within a particular area or for those who are members of a health plan or insurance fund;
- a clearer definition and delineation of the purchasing function such that responsibility is being shifted from the heartland of government to an agency or agencies, the primary responsibility of which is to purchase healthcare and obtain value for money; in Germany, for example, there is now an increased emphasis on the power of insurance schemes;
- a growing appreciation of the need for the purchasers of healthcare to manage the evolution and development of clinical practice in partnership with clinical professions;
- increasing public and political interest in the evidence on which decisions about the effectiveness and safety of healthcare are based.

As a result of these common problems, pressures and solutions, systems of health service organisation are also beginning to converge. In order to meet these powerful challenges, however, the principles of evidence-based healthcare can be applied to great effect, irrespective of whether a health service is organised nationally (as in the UK) or by province (as in Canada), whether it is tax-based or insurance-based (as in Japan), whether the main source of funding is public or private (as in the US).

References

1. GLASZIOU, P.T. and MACKERRAS, D.M. (1993) *Vitamin A supplementation in infectious diseases: a meta-analysis.* Br. Med. J. 306: 366–70.
2. GARNER, P. (1996) *Routine antimalarial drug chemoprophylaxis during pregnancy in endemic malarious areas,* in PHENG, C., GARNER, P., GELBAND, H. and SALINAS, R. (Eds) *Parasitic diseases module of the Cochrane Database of Systematic Reviews [Updated 29 February 1996].* The Cochrane Collaboration; Issue 3. Update Software, Oxford.

CONFESSIONS OF AN AMANUENSIS

Although famous for his work in electromagnetism, it is far from common knowledge that the young Michael Faraday acted as an amanuensis to Sir Humphrey Davy following an injury to Davy's eyes in a laboratory explosion.

The word 'amanuensis' was first recorded in 1619, derived from the Latin 'manu' for hand and 'ensis', a suffix meaning 'belonging to'. The definition in the *Shorter Oxford English Dictionary* is given as 'one who copies or writes from dictation'. This has been my function in the preparation of this book, which is a record of the work done during 1990–1995, principally in Oxford, to promote 'evidence-based healthcare'. In the future, this work will be a focus for the Institute of Health Sciences, Oxford.

At first, the idea of commissioning a multi-author book was considered, but rejected because of the problems inherent in such a project, particularly on a topic like evidence-based healthcare in which there is so much cross-cutting from one approach to another. It would have been extremely difficult to fuse several different contributions into a coherent whole, and therefore the decision was taken for one person to 'copy or write from dictation' from a wide variety of people. These people work in the four counties that comprised the old Oxford Regional Health Authority. They built on the original ideas of the team at McMaster University, comprising Larry Chambers, Gordon Guyatt, Brian Haynes, Jonathan Lomas, Andy Oxman and Dave Sackett, who is a source of inspiration and has helped us so much since making the bold move to emigrate to the UK.

Those whose work has been drawn upon to a considerable extent by this amanuensis are:

Clive Adams, Doug Altman, Anne Brice, Catherine Brogan, Shaun Brogan, Chris Bulstrode, Iain Chalmers, Miles Chippendale, Andy Chivers, Martin Dawes, Anna Donald, Gordon Dooley, Jayne Edwards, Jim Elliott, David Gill, Michael Goldacre, Sian Griffiths, Nick Hicks, Alison Hill, Richard Himsworth, Tony Hope, Carol Lefebvre, Mark Lodge, Steve McDonald, Ian McKinnell, Henry McQuay, Jill Meara, Ruairidh Milne, Andrew Moore, David Naylor, Gill Needham, Ian Owens, Judy Palmer, David Pencheon, William Rosenberg, Jill Sanders, Ken Schultz, Valerie Seagroatt, Mark Starr, Barbara Stocking, Martin Vessey, and Chris Williams.

Many of these people have been supported by the NHS R&D Programme and the leadership of Sir Michael Peckham was very important in the evolution of evidence-based healthcare.

I am also indebted to those people, in various teams, with whom I have worked on the development of these ideas: the GRiPP team, the CASP team, the R&D team, and those in the Cochrane Collaboration and in the IHS Library.

Simply stringing words together is only part of the preparation of a text like this; the final product has been the combined work of a small team. The team is supported by Ann Southwell, who provided the business management skills which underpinned the creation of many of the projects that contributed to the development of evidence-based healthcare. Karen McKendry was the wizard with Powerpoint who created many of the diagrams that punctuate and enliven the prose; André Tomlin provided the technical expertise to ensure that the advice on searching was accurate; without their contribution the book would have been of much poorer quality. Finally, I would like to thank the duo who hammered the raw metal into its final form: Rosemary Lees and Erica Ison. They have been endlessly good-humoured and hard-working and applied not only effort but also the highest level of skill to transform pig iron into steel, discursive prose into a text that is much briefer, clearer and more powerful than it was when it left the hand of the amanuensis.

Finally, like another Scottish amanuensis – James Boswell – I must acknowledge the burden borne by my family – Jackie, Em, and Tat – who have put up with it all.

The production of this book was supported by charitable trust funds, into which any income derived from publication shall be returned. The objective in the disbursement of monies from these funds is the promotion of epidemiology as a practical tool for all healthcare decision makers working for what the new President of the Royal Statistical Society has called the 'promotion of an evidence-based society'.[1]

Reference

1. SMITH, A.F.M. (1996) *Mad cows and Ecstasy: chance and choice in an evidence-based society.* J. R. Statist. Soc. A. 159: 367–83.

ELECTRONIC UPDATES

Between the submission of the typescript and the receipt of the page proofs, important new papers have been published and new examples of evidence-based healthcare identified; between submission of the page proofs and publication of the book the same events will recur. It is unlikely that any of these events will substantially change the book, but evidence-based healthcare is evolving and the reader of this book in a year or two's time will need more references and new tools for decision making. For this reason we have set up an Evidence-Based Healthcare Toolbox on the World Wide Web – an increasingly important source of information on healthcare, as described in a new book called *Medical Information on the Internet*.[1]

The Web site of the Evidence-Based Healthcare Toolbox is
http://www.ihs.ox.ac.uk/ebh.html
It is linked to the Evidence-Based Medicine Toolbox, primarily for clinicians, which is a complementary tool to *Evidence-Based Medicine*, the companion volume to this book, written for those making decisions about individual patients.[2]

These pages allow you the opportunity to make comments and criticisms and we look forward to hearing from you.

References

1. KILEY, R. (1996) *Medical Information on the Internet*. Churchill Livingstone, London.
2. SACKETT, D.L., RICHARDSON, W.S., ROSENBERG, W. and HAYNES, R.B. (1997) *Evidence-Based Medicine: How to Practice and Teach EBM*. Churchill Livingstone, London.

PROLOGUE 1

Dear Reader,

Empathise with the walnut. You have put it into one of those nutcrackers in which the nut is contained within a wooden cup and pressure is exerted by a wooden screw. The screw can be turned on the nut either to crack the shell and release the kernel whole or to smash the nut to smithereens.

Any health service is in the same situation as the nut: existing within a resource envelope that is subject to increasing pressure resulting from the population ageing, the advent of new technology and rising patient expectations.

Commentary

What do I mean when I refer to a health service? In this context, it represents a decision maker, i.e. those like you who will feel the pressure as the screw tightens. Each year, for every million population, millions of decisions are made about individual patients by clinicians, and thousands of decisions are made about groups of patients or populations. This book has been written for those who have to make decisions about groups of patients or populations. A companion book on evidence-based medicine is aimed primarily at clinicians, but the essence of this discipline has been distilled in Chapter 9 because decisions about individual patients and those about groups are inter-related. Clinicians who are also managers or involved in managing will benefit from developing the skills described in both books because, although concepts, such as appropriateness or effectiveness, are the same, a different perspective needs to be brought to bear in each sphere.

CHAPTER 1

EVIDENCE-BASED HEALTHCARE

1.1 THE ETERNAL VERITIES: EVIDENCE, VALUES AND RESOURCES

Decisions about groups of patients or populations are made by combining three factors:

1. evidence;
2. values;
3. resources.

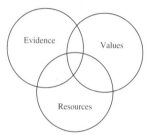

At present, many healthcare decisions are based principally on values and resources – opinion-based decision making; little attention has been given or is paid to evidence derived from research – the scientific factor. This will change: as the pressure on resources increases, decisions will have to be made explicitly and publicly; those who take decisions will need to be able to produce and describe the evidence on which each decision was based. Even in cases for which evidence is difficult to find or poor in quality, the decision maker must search for it, appraise and present it, even if the decision taken may ultimately be dominated by values and resources. Thus, as the pressure on resources increases, there will be a transition from opinion-based decision making to evidence-based decision making.

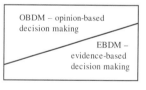

1.2 EVIDENCE-BASED DECISION MAKING

In the 21st century, the healthcare decision maker, that is, anyone who makes decisions about groups of patients or populations, will have to practise evidence-based decision making. Every decision will have to be based on a systematic appraisal of the best evidence available (Fig. 1.1). To accomplish this, the best available evidence relating to a particular decision must be found.

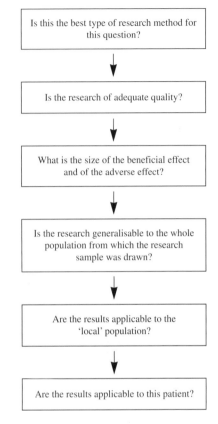

Fig. 1.1
Asking the right questions

The skills required of a practising evidence-based decision maker are:

- an ability to define criteria such as effectiveness, safety and acceptability;
- an ability to find articles on the effectiveness, safety and acceptability of a new test or treatment;
- an ability to assess the quality of evidence;
- an ability to assess whether the results of research are generalisable to the whole population from which the sample was drawn;
- an ability to assess whether the results of the research are applicable to the 'local' population.

It may seem ambitious to predicate the development of such skills, but there is evidence that it can be done. Indeed, to assume that healthcare decision makers can operate in any other way in the hard times ahead is unrealistic.

In the past, healthcare managers have tended to focus on cost and quality, that is, with 'doing things right', and to leave 'doing the right things' to other forces and chance. This situation can no longer continue. Everyone involved in decision making must have the skills to enable them to make decisions about 'doing the right things'. All chief executives should be able to discriminate between a good and a bad systematic review; directors of finance should be able to find and appraise studies on health service cost-effectiveness; any medical director should be able to determine whether a randomised controlled trial in a specialty other than their own is biased. These are the management skills necessary for the provision of healthcare in the 21st century.

1.3 EVIDENCE-BASED HEALTHCARE – A SCIENTIFIC APPROACH TO HEALTHCARE MANAGEMENT

Over the last two decades, tremendous advances have been made in the health sciences. Hitherto these advances have principally been used to help clinicians, such that clinical decision making is now based on information derived from research to a much greater degree than it was. This practice is called evidence-based medicine or evidence-based clinical practice (a more generic term).

In this book, readers will be shown how some of the scientific advances and methods that have underpinned the development of clinical practice can also underpin decision making involving the care of groups of patients and of populations. Evidence-based healthcare is a discipline centred upon evidence-based decision making about individual patients, groups of patients or populations, which may be manifest as evidence-based purchasing or evidence-based management.

The science of most relevance to healthcare decision making is epidemiology, that is, the study of disease in groups of patients and populations. Although other sciences, such as occupational psychology, can be a source of information for managers, epidemiology is the foundation of healthcare management.

1.4 THE GROWING NEED FOR EVIDENCE-BASED HEALTHCARE

The need and the demand for healthcare are increasing. In almost every country, the rate of growth of both need and demand for healthcare is faster than the rate of increase in resources available for providing it. There are four main reasons for this, which are described below (see also Fig. 1.2 in which the interaction of these factors is shown).

1. Population ageing

Population ageing is the single most important factor increasing the need for healthcare. As the number of older people increases, so does the need for healthcare.

In addition, the interaction of an ageing population and rising patient expectations is significant. Cohorts of individuals currently becoming old will have different expectations from those who are already old. In future, older people will be better organised, more assertive and have higher expectations, both of the quality of health that they wish to enjoy (75-year-olds will not accept chest pain as an inevitable consequence of biological ageing) and of the quality and volume of health services to which they are entitled.

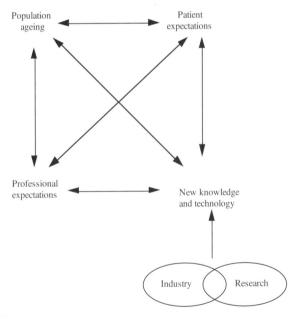

Fig. 1.2

An ageing population will also have an impact on professional expectations and behaviour. Furthermore, professionals in some specialties may have to alter their orientation to reflect the changing demography and need for healthcare services. In dentistry, for example, the care of older people will become a major source of work.

Developments in new technology will also be influenced by population ageing. It is inappropriate to think of 'care of the elderly' and 'high-technology medicine' as mutually exclusive or alternatives competing for funding. Many of the new technological developments are beneficial to older people and will be used by them; for example, radiotherapy treatment for cancer. Consequently, the impact and cost of population ageing must be considered not only in the context of geriatric or social services but also in relation to the effects those factors will have on services using new and expensive technology. Coronary artery bypass grafting is an example of 'high-technology' healthcare that is now a commonly performed operation in old age, and the average age of people receiving their first or follow-up grafts is increasing; an increase in the number of older people will mean an increase in the demand for coronary artery bypass grafting, irrespective of the trends in the incidence and prevalence of coronary heart disease.

2. New technology and knowledge

New technologies will continue to be developed by industry and research workers within health services and related disciplines.

The nature of the technology may be either 'high' – for instance, making use of biomaterials, utilising the results of sophisticated basic research or computer systems or a combination of all three – or 'low ', for example, effective simple interventions to prevent postnatal depression. Research findings indicate what it is possible to achieve, which will then influence both patient and professional expectations.

Sometimes, the application of a new technology will result in lower healthcare costs or in lower costs elsewhere in the economy, but even if healthcare costs are ultimately reduced by the use of a new technology there is often an increase in cost in the short term.

Moreover, effective new technology increases the need for healthcare if 'need' is defined as a health problem for which there is an effective intervention. When an effective intervention has been developed, a previously insoluble problem is transformed into a health need for which there is a concomitant claim on resources. The knowledge that such an effective intervention exists leads to public and professional demand for that service to be provided. If a false impression of effectiveness is given, this may lead to an inappropriate demand: for example, the discovery of specific genes for the development of breast cancer has precipitated a demand for counselling services, but as yet there is no evidence that a woman being aware of the fact that she has a breast cancer gene or genes is beneficial unless that woman is willing to undergo bilateral mastectomy.

3. Patient expectations

Patient expectations of healthcare are rising, reflecting societal changes in attitude towards the provision of goods and services, a trend usually called 'consumerism'.

There is general acceptance that the enjoyment of good health is a desirable and achievable objective; thus, if people have an expectation that their health should be better than it is, they will seek out services they believe will improve their health.

In most developed countries, this trend includes rising expectations of the accessibility and quality of services, and of the accountability of service providers should there be any failure in the quality of healthcare. People expect:

- easy access to services;
- high-quality services;
- redress and compensation should there be a failure of service or, in some cases, a perceived failure of service.

All these factors of themselves will increase the demand for healthcare, but rising patient expectations are also fuelled by the development of new technology. Changing attitudes, especially in those becoming elderly, will mean that the sector of society which has the greatest need for healthcare will also make more demands in the future than it has in the past.

4. Professional expectations

Professional expectations and attitudes are influenced by patient expectations. If patients who are 90 years old seek hip replacements, this will affect professional attitudes and expectations about the services that should be offered. Changing patient expectations about healthcare and the quality of healthcare may also influence professional attitudes and behaviour in a negative way: the threat of litigation may stimulate an increase in the practice of 'defensive medicine'.

Professional expectations are also influenced by developments in technology in that any new developments serve as a stimulus to increase expectations. An important managerial challenge for the future will be to help professionals be more critical in their appraisal of new technology and to change the paradigm of healthcare such that a large proportion of the interventions offered to the population are those that have been shown by the performance of good-quality research to be effective.

1.5 BARRIERS TO GOOD DECISION MAKING

The performance of an individual or team is a function of, that is, it is determined by, three variables: it is *directly* related to the level of *motivation* and the *competence* of the individual, and *inversely* related to the *barriers* the individual has to overcome in order to perform well.

$$P = \frac{M \times C}{B}$$

where P = performance
       M = motivation
       C = competence
       B = barriers

My overall purpose in writing this book is twofold:

1. to improve the competence of decision makers;
2. to strengthen any decision maker's motivation to use scientific methods when making a decision.

However, it is also necessary to outline the barriers that any decision maker has to overcome or, to express the converse, the resources every decision maker requires in order to be able to practise evidence-based decision making (see Box 1.1).

It is also vital for any decision maker intent upon evidence-based decision making to be working in an environment in which appropriate and effective decision making is encouraged, that is, an organisation committed to evidence-based decision making (Chapter 7).

Box 1.1   Resources necessary to every decision maker

- The support of a librarian
- Access to The Cochrane Library, MEDLINE, EMBASE and HealthSTAR (Appendix I)
- Access to the World Wide Web
- Access to a personal computer with reference management software so that any articles identified as appropriate for use as evidence can be stored systematically

1.6   DEFINING THE SCOPE OF EVIDENCE-BASED HEALTHCARE

Evidence-based healthcare consists of three main stages, as illustrated in Fig. 1.3.

1. Producing evidence
Producing evidence is the responsibility of research workers. In general, research is conducted in one of two contexts:

- within a framework set by decision makers, when research is commissioned by governments or research councils;

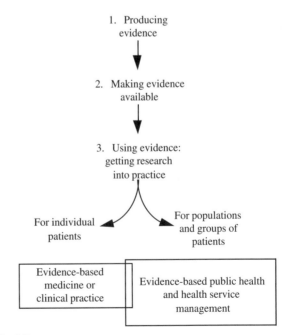

Fig. 1.3

- within a subject area, or on a topic, determined by the researcher(s) who will then seek funding from a charity or other body; the funding body will support that research project if it is of good quality – responsive funding.

2. Making evidence available

Making the evidence derived from research available is vital because otherwise the potential value of that new knowledge will never be realised. If research evidence has been made available, it is possible to gain access to it. In this book, examples are given of ways in which individuals can access information in libraries and from databases such as MEDLINE, although better systems for gaining access to information at the time it is needed, on a ward round, in a surgery or in a patient's own home, must be developed.

3. Using evidence

There are two main ways in which research evidence can be used:

- to improve clinical practice (see Section 1.6.1);
- to improve health service management (see Section 1.6.2).

1.6.1 Evidence-based clinical practice

Evidence-based clinical practice is an approach to decision making in which the clinician uses the best evidence available, in consultation with the patient, to decide upon the option which suits that patient best. Evidence-based clinical practice is described briefly in Chapter 9, particularly from the perspective of the health service manager who can do much to promote both evidence-based clinical practice and evidence-based patient choice.

1.6.2 Evidence-based policy making, purchasing and management for health services

Managers who are responsible for health services for groups of patients or populations have to make many decisions, all of which will fall into one of three main categories:

1. policy;
2. purchasing;
3. management.

As the number of constraints around decision making increase, all three categories of decision will need to be based on evidence. The contents of this book will help health service personnel who have to make decisions about policy, purchasing and management develop the skills necessary to base those decisions on the best evidence available.

1. Policy decisions

Policy making is a political process: it is based not only on evidence but also on the value politicians place upon different types of decision making, for example, whether centralised as opposed to decentralised decision making is favoured.

Certain policy decisions might result in changes to the financing of a health service and to the way in which that service is organised to account for the resources used. In the UK, the introduction of the purchaser/provider split changed the financial responsibility and authority of both purchasers and providers, and the introduction of GP fundholding changed the way in which finance flowed in the National Health Service (NHS), a change that also altered the authority and responsibility of those professionals working in any general practice which became fundholding.

2. Purchasing decisions

Purchasing is a process by which those responsible for expenditure on healthcare for a population or group of patients enter into a set of contracts with the providers of health services to obtain the delivery of particular services at a specified level of quality and an agreed cost. Purchasers may be public bodies, such as a health authority, as is the case in the UK, or private organisations, e.g. insurance companies, as is the case in the Netherlands (but it should be noted that insurance companies in many countries are supported by the state, provided certain requirements have been met). If finance is limited, purchasing is often linked to prioritisation.

3. Management decisions

Management is the process whereby the resources allocated to healthcare expenditure for a particular population or group of patients are utilised to best effect.

1.6.3 'Managed care'

In the past, it was possible to distinguish between two types of healthcare: clinical practice and public health (for the dichotomies between the two, see Table 1.1).

Table 1.1

Clinical care	Public health
For individuals	For populations
Treatment for those who feel ill	Treatment of those who feel well
Low NNT	High NNT
Decisions unique to the individual	Decisions common to populations
Difficult to produce systems and guidelines	Easy to produce systems and guidelines
Paradigm problem: a patient who is feeling weak and tired	Paradigm problem: a population at risk of polio

Nowadays, however, this sharp distinction no longer obtains, and increasing effort is being invested into managing in a standard way the care of patients who suffer from the same condition; this is known as managed care. Managed care lies between clinical practice and public health on the spectrum of healthcare.

Clinical care	Managed care	Public health

Within a managed care system, standard care is delivered to groups of patients who have certain common conditions for which it is possible to define a core set of interventions and services which those suffering from that condition should receive.

As the application of managed care has sometimes resulted in a greater involvement of nurses in clinical decision making, either when offering a point of primary contact or when ensuring that a proposed referral to a specialised service is appropriate, the need for diagnostic and treatment algorithms has also increased.

At first sight, it may seem as if the introduction of managed care will counteract the vagaries of clinical practice and facilitate the introduction of evidence-based healthcare. However, although managed care has an important contribution to make, for instance, by reducing the duration of hospital stay or increasing the proportion of heart attack patients who are prescribed beta-blocker drugs, it should not be regarded as a universal panacea for healthcare problems for the following reasons:

- Some patients may present with problems that will not allow them to be slotted into a managed care system.
- Patients whom it is possible to treat within a managed care system, because they have a disease such as diabetes or asthma, may have individual characteristics that make it difficult to apply the guidelines to all aspects of care.
- The detailed control of decision making inherent in a managed care system may cause clinicians to become disaffected such that they perform less well in another sphere of clinical practice, such as communication with the patient.

The development of managed care does, however, offer important opportunities in the introduction of evidence-based healthcare (see Appendix VD).

1.7 THE LIMITATIONS OF EVIDENCE-BASED HEALTHCARE

The practice of evidence-based healthcare enables those managing health services to determine the mix of services and procedures that will give the greatest benefit to the population served by that health service. However, there is no guarantee that any potential benefits identified within a research setting will be realised in practice, because outcome is also determined by the quality of management. To ensure that a population/group of patients receives the maximum health benefit at the lowest possible risk and cost from the resources available, both evidence-based healthcare and quality management are essential practices (Table 1.2).

Evidence-based healthcare + quality management
=
maximum health benefit at lowest risk and cost

Table 1.2

Managerial responsibility	Managerial action
Ensure that all the services and procedures are supported by high-quality evidence, and they do more good than harm	Technology assessment; critical appraisal
Ensure that the mix of services and procedures is that which will give the greatest benefit for the population served	Needs assessment; priority setting; decision making
Ensure that services and clinical practice are of sufficiently high quality to realise the potential for health improvement demonstrated in research settings	Professional education; public education; purchasing; quality management; clinical audit

1.8 THE LIMITS OF HEALTHCARE

The best healthcare is that:

- from which, based on the best evidence available, all ineffective interventions have been eliminated;
- in which the interventions undertaken are of the highest possible effectiveness for those groups of patients within the population most likely to benefit;
- in which all services are delivered at the highest possible quality.

However, the health of a population is determined by four factors, only one of which is healthcare. The other three factors are:

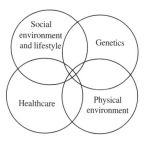

- physical environment;
- social environment and lifestyle;
- genetics – an individual's genotype may confer a degree of protection or susceptibility to factors in the environment, whether physical or social, that trigger disease.

Thus, even the provision of the best healthcare will not necessarily ensure optimum levels of health in a population.

Sick individuals present to clinicians with complicated problems which require an appreciation of the relationship between disease and illness.

The terms 'disease' and 'illness' are sometimes used interchangeably, but they have distinct meanings, as the definitions in the *Shorter Oxford English Dictionary* demonstrate.

> 'Disease: a condition of the body, or of some part or organ of the body, in which its functions are disturbed or deranged.'
>
> 'Illness: bad or unhealthy condition of the body (or, formerly, of a part); the condition of being ill.'

A disease is a condition from which an individual suffers, like tuberculosis; an illness is a state of being, in which the individual enjoys the privileges of illness but must obey certain rules (see Table 1.3)

Table 1.3

The privileges of illness	The rules of illness
Being excused normal social duties	The patient must be seen to be trying to get better
Extra sympathy and attention	The patient must give up many normal social pleasures, e.g. going out to parties

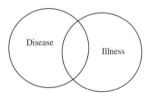

The relationship between disease and illness is best shown in a Venn diagram. Most people who have a disease are also ill, although the degree to which any individual claims the privileges of illness varies considerably from one person to another. Some people have a disease but are not ill: an individual with undiagnosed diabetes has a disease but is unaware of the change in social status that will pertain when the diagnosis is known. Some people who have a disease do not wish to be ill or to be treated in a special way, a characteristic of people who have disabilities but do not wish to be discriminated against simply because of a disability resulting from disease.

There are also people who feel ill but in whom no causal disease can be found to explain their symptoms. This type of disorder has two common manifestations:

1. medically unexplained physical symptoms (MUPS), sometimes called somatoform disorders or somatisation, usually pain of various types;
2. hypochondriasis or excessive anxiety about a disease, usually cancer.

These disorders are very common.

One estimate is that about half of all those people attending general medicine out-patient clinics have MUPS.[1] MUPS are reactions to various forms of external strain that may occur:

- as an alternative to constructive adaptive behaviour that will remove or reduce the causal strain;
- as an unproductive substitute for effective coping, as shown in Fig. 1.4.

There is, however, important evidence that MUPS can be treated effectively with cognitive therapy.[1] Indeed, as the pressure on resources increases, it will be necessary to treat this large group of patients in a more systematic manner: for example, at present, a woman presenting with pelvic pain may be referred to as many as three different clinics and

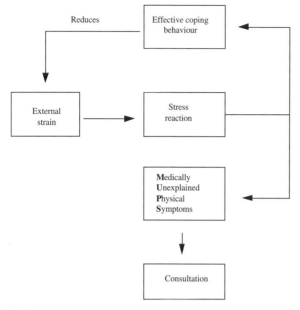

Fig. 1.4

have various doctors in training in different specialties applying endoscopic and laparoscopic interventions on separate occasions in an attempt to cure the pain. Following a short course of cognitive behavioural therapy, it was found that such patients experienced a higher recovery rate.[1] This paper is important: it shows that it is possible to apply randomised controlled trial methodology to such subtle and complex problems as MUPS.

The authors of a paper on somatisation and medicalisation in the era of managed care[2] argue that the rate of presentation of MUPS will increase as managed care becomes more prevalent in the USA. It is encouraging to note that some of the factors identified in that article as leading to increased referral rates are not relevant in the UK, where there has been a form of managed care, namely, capitation-based general practice, since the inception of the NHS. Nonetheless, MUPS is a common problem in primary care.

References

1. SPECKENS, A.E.M., van HEMERT, A.M., SPINHOVEN, P. et al. (1995) *Cognitive behavioural therapy for medically unexplained physical sypmtoms: a randomised controlled trial.* Br. Med. J. 311: 1328–32.
2. BARSKY, A.J. and BORUS, J.F. (1995) *Somatization and medicalization in the era of managed care.* JAMA 274: 1931–4.

PROLOGUE 2

Dear Reader,

Empathise with the purchaser. He felt gutted. He read with dismay the business case that the Trust had put together to support the acquisition of spiral computed tomography (CT) which had revenue consequences of about £500 000 a year for several years. How could they? They knew their main purchaser faced a financial problem – a matter of a few millions. The Trust itself had a financial gap to close between their prices and the purchaser's position. Purchaser and provider had been discussing this gap 'maturely' for weeks, or so the purchaser thought, but of spiral CT nary a mention. Now it pops up like a jack-in-a-bloody-box.

Dear Reader,

Empathise with the provider. She felt gutted. The purchaser had said they couldn't support the acquisition of new spiral CT kit. It was standard now; every Trust had it. They would be virtually the only Trust without it, and the business case was good. When compared with ordinary CT, the images are more accurate, disease can be diagnosed earlier and the scanning time is much faster, which makes it more acceptable to patients. It would increase the productivity of the Trust and reduce waiting times; surely the purchaser had been demanding all these things from them for months. Now they turn round and say it's no go.

Commentary

The prologue presents a seemingly intractable situation of irreconcilable differences. To resolve the conflict, both parties need to find and appraise the evidence on which claim and counterclaim are based and then discuss the quality of the evidence, the size of the effect suggested by that evidence and the applicability of those research findings to the population being served. This approach will be increasingly required as those who make decisions are subject to increasing pressure to 'do the right things right'.

CHAPTER 2

'DOING THE RIGHT THINGS RIGHT'

2.1 THE EVOLUTION OF EVIDENCE-BASED HEALTHCARE (FIG. 2.1)

2.1.1 Doing things cheaper

During the 1970s, financial pressure began to mount in the NHS after two decades during which investment in healthcare had increased steadily. The OPEC crisis and its financial consequences initiated an era in which healthcare decision makers became more cost conscious. They were exhorted to increase efficiency, although this was actually manifest as an increase in productivity. Productivity is the relationship between inputs and outputs [e.g. number of bed days (therefore money necessary) per operation],

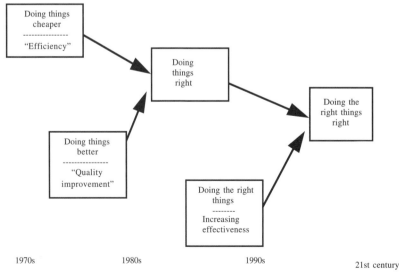

Fig. 2.1
The evolution of evidence-based healthcare

whereas efficiency is the relationship between inputs and outcomes [e.g. number of bed days (therefore money necessary) to obtain 1 extra year of life]. Unfortunately, the two words are often used synonymously (see Sections 6.6.1.1 and 6.6.1.2).

The impetus was to reduce cost per case by ensuring that healthcare was delivered for the shortest time, in the least expensive place, by the least expensive professional, using the cheapest possible drugs or equipment sufficient to ensure effectiveness and safety.

2.1.2 Doing things better

During the 1980s, although the demand for increased efficiency was maintained, there was a new imperative, that of delivering quality improvement. As patients became better informed, more assertive and better organised, their expectations increased. Patients expected:

- easier access to services;
- more effective healthcare;
- safer care;
- more information;
- better communication.

These expectations for the provision of better healthcare reflected the general societal trend towards 'consumerism'. The response within health services was 'to do things better' using the tools of quality assurance and clinical audit.

2.1.3 Doing things right

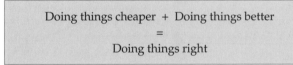

Doing things cheaper + Doing things better
=
Doing things right

During the 1970s and 1980s, health service managers concentrated on 'doing things right'. Unfortunately, 'doing things right' is only half of the old management adage; the other half is 'doing the right things'.

2.1.4 Doing the right things

In healthcare, the overall objective is to do more good than harm. However, it is always important to remember that virtually all interventions have the potential to harm.

The interventions delivered within a health service can be categorised into three types according to their impact on patients:

1. doing more good than harm;
2. doing more harm than good;
3. of unknown effect.

The phrase 'more good than harm' encompasses four important concepts, three of which are obvious by virtue of their representation in words while the fourth is unwritten.

> **'good'** – this term implies effectiveness but also includes safety and acceptability (see Sections 6.3 and 6.4);
> **'harm'** – this aspect of care should always be sought by decision makers. Product champions who argue for a new service or intervention to be introduced usually concentrate on the good the innovation will do. Even in cases where the possibility of harm is acknowledged, professionals may place a lower value on harm than the potential recipients of a service (see Section 9.3.1);
> **'more'** – although the definition of 'more' may be self-evident, the magnitude of any difference described by the term is as important as the existence of a difference. It is also important to bear in mind that the magnitude of any difference observed in a research study, and sometimes its existence, is determined by:

- the efficacy of the intervention when administered by the best hands in a research setting;
- the quality of the service in which the intervention is actually delivered (Table 2.1).

Table 2.1

Quality of service	Balance
Very high	Good much greater than harm
Average	Good greater than harm
Below average	Good and harm equally balanced
Very low	Harm greater than good

> The unwritten factor is the **strength of the evidence**, which is determined by the quality of the research on which the evidence is based (see Chapter 5). The proposition that a therapy or test does more good than harm should be discarded if it is only an expression of personal opinion but it should be used as evidence if it is a conclusion drawn from the conduct of high-quality

research, the results of which showed that the intervention made a substantial difference with a low probability that the results were due to chance or biased findings.

Once the balance of good to harm has been established, decision makers then need information on the costs of different options.

2.2 THE NEW MANAGEMENT AGENDA: 'DOING THE RIGHT THINGS RIGHT'

This book has as a focus evidence-based decision making, that is, how decision makers can search for, appraise and use evidence. However, few health service management texts or courses appear to address the particular context of a health service, namely, a service driven not only by science but also by decentralised decision making – clinicians make many of the decisions thereby determining service provision and resource expenditure. Given this context, it is of paramount importance that those who make decisions about healthcare base those decisions on good evidence, using as a framework the classification of healthcare interventions set out in Section 2.1.4 (see also Table 2.2).

The evidence-based approach to the delivery of health services initiates a new management agenda:

• the initiation of strategies to increase the good:harm ratio (Table 2.2);
• the promotion of change in clinical practice;
• the acceleration of change in clinical practice (see Section 9.5);
• the promotion of research.

Table 2.2

Type of intervention	Strategies to increase the good:harm ratio
Does more good than harm	• Promote use if it is affordable • Take steps to increase good and decrease harm to make ratio more favourable – quality improvement
Does more harm than good	• Stop them starting • Stop them if it is not possible to increase good and decrease harm sufficiently to convert them into type A interventions
Of unknown effect	• Stop them starting • Promote the conduct of RCTs both for new interventions and for interventions already in practice

In most health services operating today, the distribution of the various types of interventions administered probably follows that shown in Fig. 2.2.

The optimal distribution of interventions administered is represented in Fig. 2.3.

Although quality improvement and cost reduction have been the imperatives in health service management since the 1980s, the other activities shown in Table 2.2, which will

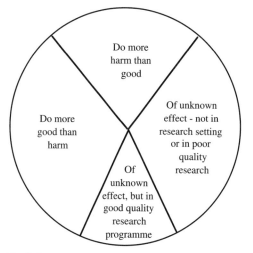

Fig. 2.2
Present distribution of the various types of intervention

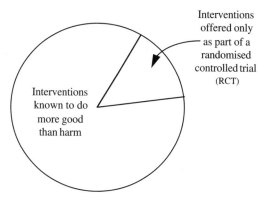

Fig. 2.3
Optimal distribution of interventions

have an influence on not only *how* clinicians practise but *what* they practise, are new items on the agenda.

2.2.1 Strategies that increase the good:harm ratio

It may take years for an effective intervention to be mentioned, much less promoted, in a textbook. The classic example is that of a study by Antman et al[1] of the delay in recommending thrombolysis as an effective intervention following myocardial infarction (see Fig. 2.4). This example demonstrates that even when information is available, implementation is often slow and sporadic.

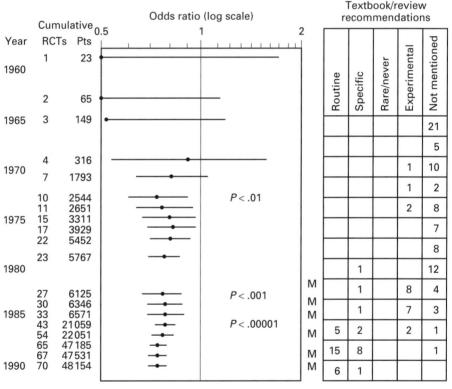

Fig. 2.4
Thrombolytic therapy: delay between evidence of effectiveness of the intervention appearing and its inclusion in textbooks (Source: Antman et al[1], JAMA, 8 July 1992, vol 268, p. 242. Copyright 1992, American Medical Association)

Some clinicians believe delay in implementation to be a virtue, often citing as justification for their stance the consequences of the administration of thalidomide as a hypnotic to pregnant women. However, the key to control lies not in delaying the implementation of research findings but in the critical appraisal of the best research evidence available and sound decision making based on that appraisal. In fact, the use of thalidomide is an example of the failure to base decisions on good evidence.

If there is evidence that an intervention does more good than harm and that intervention is affordable, decision makers must manage its introduction within the health service (see Section 7.1.7). This will require appropriate professional training and patient education to promote good decision making, and the development of systems of care supported by quality standards and mechanisms for the detection and correction of quality failures. All these steps are necessary to ensure good clinical outcomes.

> Good clinical decision making + good systems
> =
> good clinical outcomes

If interventions are of unproven efficacy or are doing more harm than good, decision makers must ensure that either they are not introduced – 'stop them starting' – or, if they have already been introduced, that they are no longer practised – 'start stopping them'.

Action to prevent the initiation or continuation of harmful interventions can be taken through:

- public education, for instance, about the benefits of aspirin after acute myocardial infarction (AMI);
- professional training, for instance, to promote the benefits of thrombolysis;
- purchasing; for instance, to specify in contracts the standard of delivery of thrombolysis treatment expected for patients with AMI (door-to-needle time);
- audit, in which performance is measured against a specified standard.

2.2.2   Managing the evolution of clinical practice

It is important to manage the introduction of any change in clinical practice; it is no longer sustainable to allow clinicians to make decisions about such changes in isolation. Although clinicians do implement changes in clinical practice that improve health, some of which will be achievable at a reasonable or reduced cost, they do not invariably choose 'the right things to do'. For example, the intervention known as laparoscopic cholecystectomy underwent rapid and widespread introduction in health services throughout the world at the instigation of clinicians before high-quality evidence of its efficacy was available. The publication of the results of an RCT of laparoscopic cholecystectomy subsequently showed there was little benefit associated with the procedure.[2] Sometimes changes in clinical practice can worsen outcomes overall; for instance, changes in the prescription of antibiotics have contributed to the genesis of a modern epidemic, the evolution of antibiotic-resistant bacteria, which has resulted in an increase in health service costs and in mortality.

Until now, the evolution of clinical practice has been piecemeal and unco-ordinated, driven by individual clinicians. This situation is no longer acceptable and those responsible for the management and funding of health services must develop a new relationship within which clinicians (collectively) and managers can work together to guide the course of the evolution of clinical practice. This is probably the most challenging item on the new management agenda.

2.2.3 Promoting trials

If the intervention is of unknown effect, it should not be introduced, or if it is already in service it should be withdrawn until its effects have been investigated: within an RCT to determine the beneficial effects (Section 5.3) and within a case-control or cohort study to identify any adverse effects (Sections 5.4 and 5.5). It is possible to promote the performance of trials not only by creating a culture in which interventions of unknown efficacy have to be evaluated scientifically from the first patient but also by ensuring that those responsible for any health service invest in research and development.

References

1. ANTMAN, E.M., LAU, J., KUPELNICK, B. et al. (1992) *A comparison of results of meta-analysis of randomized controlled trials and recommendations of clinical experts.* JAMA 268: 240-8.
2. MAJEED, A.W., TROY, G., NICHOLL, J.P. et al. (1996) *Randomised, prospective single blind comparison of laparoscopic versus small incision cholecystectomy.* Lancet 347: 989-94.

2.3 THE IMPACT OF SCIENCE ON CLINICAL PRACTICE AND HEALTHCARE COSTS

As a scientific approach to healthcare decision making is championed in this book, it is appropriate to describe the impact new technology is having on health services worldwide.

Healthcare costs are increased by many factors (see Fig. 2.5):

* population ageing;
* changes in the volume and intensity of clinical practice;
* medical price inflation;
* general price inflation.

The ways in which changes or innovations in clinical practice increase the cost of care are manifold (see Box 2.1).

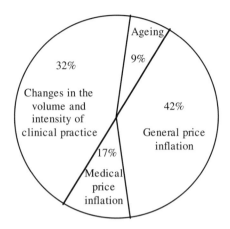

Fig. 2.5
Factors contributing to the increase in healthcare costs

Box 2.1   How innovations in clinical practice increase costs

- Treating conditions that were previously untreatable.
- Treating people who would previously have been untreated because of changing professional perceptions of need and appropriateness and changing public expectations. These may result from:
  – increasing safety of intervention;
  – more acceptable, less invasive, more pleasant interventions;
  – changing attitudes to chronological age as a reason for refusing treatment;
  – changing expectations about health and disease.
- Providing more expensive types of treatment:
  – more expensive drugs;
  – more expensive imaging;
  – more expensive tests;
  – more expensive staff.
- More intensive clinical practice:
  – longer duration of stay;
  – more tests per patient;
  – more professional interventions per patient;
  – more treatments per patient.

Sometimes, science may be put into practice by a single, well-considered national policy decision – for example, in the UK the introduction of breast cancer screening. However, most science is introduced into clinical practice by clinicians, who then seek the resources to fund it from those who pay for the service to be delivered. A study by Eddy in the USA showed that, in a healthcare system in which expenditure is not finite, changes in the 'volume and intensity' of clinical practice are the main factors driving increases in the cost of care that can be controlled by health service managers;[1] the other causes of increasing costs are beyond the power of health service managers to control (see Fig. 2.5).

In other healthcare systems in which decisions are made within a context of finite resources, expenditure does not spiral out of control, although changes in the volume and intensity of clinical practice will generate financial and service pressures and can also drive the service in directions other than those that have been identified as priorities.

Much attention and money has been invested to ensure that clinicians 'do things right', by encouraging the performance of clinical audit, for instance. However, clinicians do not necessarily always 'do the right things'. For all healthcare professionals, but particularly clinicians, the important question to address as the next century approaches is not only 'Are we doing things right? ' or 'Are we doing the right things? ' but:

'Are we doing the right things right?'

Reference

1. EDDY, D.M. (1993) *Three battles to watch in the 1990s.* JAMA 270: 520–6.

CHAPTER 3

MAKING DECISIONS ABOUT HEALTH SERVICES

In this chapter, the focus is on the different types of intervention that can be provided within health services. When considering the issue about which a decision must be made, the decision maker needs to:

- examine the evidence put forward by the proposer of the service;
- find other evidence if it exists;
- appraise the quality of the research evidence (Chapter 5);
- estimate the effects, both beneficial and adverse, of the innovation (Chapter 6).

The nature of any problem a decision maker may face can vary in complexity. Instances of the simplest type of decision are those in which an enthusiast wishes to introduce a new treatment, service or test and the decision maker has to consider the effects of the innovation proposed. There are, however, many other decisions which are more complex; for example, the need to find efficiency savings or to reorganise a service because a lead consultant retires or some equipment needs to be replaced.

3.1 THERAPY

3.1.1 Dimensions and definitions

A therapy is any intervention given with the objective of improving the health status of patients or of populations. Drugs and surgical operations are examples of therapy but so too are preventive interventions, such as immunisation programmes or health promotion initiatives. Screening, a combination of a diagnostic test and a therapy, is discussed in Section 3.3.

The criteria used to assess a therapy are:

- effectiveness (Section 6.3);
- safety (Section 6.4);
- patient acceptability and satisfaction (Section 6.5);
- cost-effectiveness (Section 6.6);
- appropriateness (Section 6.8).

3.1.2 Searching

Good advice on searching for research evidence pertaining to a therapy was given in the ACP Journal Club.[1]

A MEDLINE search has four main components (see Table 3.1).

Table 3.1 Components of a MEDLINE search for a therapy

Component	Example
The clinical problem	Migraine
The therapy	Behaviour therapy
Study design	Review or RCT
The time frame	1985 to the present

The clinical problem is usually easy to specify.

The therapy is more difficult to specify because the thesaurus the indexers use for a therapy is not as well developed as that relating to the clinical problem; it is sometimes helpful to 'explode' the term chosen to be more inclusive and to group all the subtypes of therapy.

The study design can also be indexed under the publication type.

- The best single term to use when searching for publications from 1990 onwards is 'clinical trial'.
- As there is no specific term to search for systematic review, the term 'review' should be used.

See Appendix I for information on subject specialist databases.

3.1.3 Appraisal

In general, there are two questions that have to be asked when appraising research.

1. Is the design of this research study the most appropriate to answer my question?
2. How good is the quality of this particular research when compared with the best design of its type?

Detailed advice on appraising the quality of research and the outcomes chosen is given in Chapters 5 and 6, respectively. In this section, general advice is given on appropriate research methods for the evaluation of a therapy or an intervention designed to increase the effectiveness of a change in health service delivery.

3.1.3.1   The balance of good and harm

The randomised controlled trial (RCT) is the best method for assessing the effectiveness of a therapy (Section 5.3), in the form of either an individual trial or a systematic review of trials. However, even this powerful research method may not answer the question: 'Does this intervention do more good than harm?'.

Harmful effects of therapy (side-effects) are usually rarer than beneficial effects. Thus, a study that has been designed with sufficient power to detect a 5% improvement in the effectiveness of a new therapy when compared with an existing therapy may not be sufficiently powerful to detect any side-effects that may occur with a frequency of 1 in 1000. If the side-effect is mild, a skin rash, for example, this matters little, but if the side-effect is death this is serious. Thus, RCTs designed to assess effectiveness often need to be complemented by cohort studies to assess safety (see Section 5.5). These two types of evidence allow a purchaser or clinician to assess the balance between good and harm conferred by a therapy.

3.1.3.2   Assessing innovations in health service policy and management

The term 'intervention' usually refers to a specific therapeutic act which a professional administers to or performs on either a single patient or all the individuals in a certain 'population'. However, it is also possible to apply the term to more complicated situations in which the effects of more than one intervention are tested, for example:

- a comparison of treatment by different professionals, e.g. doctor *vs* nurse, chiropractor *vs* orthopaedic surgeon;
- a comparison of treatment by different teams within a clinical service;
- a comparison of treatment by different types of clinical service.

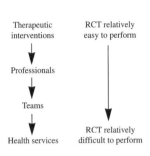

This increasing complexity of interventions, from the application of a single therapy to that of whole services, is shown in Fig. 3.1.

Although RCTs are the 'gold standard' for evaluating the effects of a therapy, they are more difficult to organise with increasing complexity of intervention, either technically, because the number of services randomly allocated may be too few to ensure the trial has adequate power, or politically, because the politicians may be reluctant to admit that a new policy should be subject to a trial – trials indicate equipoise and uncertainty.

Consequently, studies of health service organisation and delivery are sometimes investigated using research methods other than the RCT, notably:

- the cohort study (see Section 5.5);
- the case-control study (see Section 5.4).

Often, these methods require the analysis of large databases of health service utilisation.

The use of these methods allows the following types of question to be addressed.

- What is the total mortality resulting from an operation, as distinct from the mortality observed in hospital?

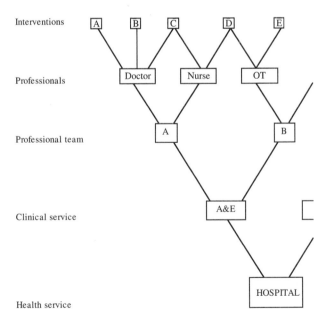

Fig. 3.1

- Is the outcome of care observed at one hospital or one type of hospital better than that which would be expected by chance?

If the mortality rate observed at one type of hospital is greater than that at another type this may indicate the need to change policy or the management of the hospital system. If the mortality rate at one hospital is greater than that at other hospitals of the same type, this may indicate a problem with quality of service delivery at that particular hospital (Section 6.7).

3.1.4 Getting research into practice

Although there has been much discussion about the problems of implementing research evidence of the effectiveness of any new intervention within the health service due to the difficulty of influencing professional practice, this type of change is relatively simple because good-quality evidence is available and should dominate decision making.

However, as the subject of the decision changes from simple interventions, such as the administration of new drugs, to more complex interventions, such as changing the patterns of skill mix or of hospital provision (see Fig. 3.1), the availability of evidence decreases, not only in absolute but also in relative terms, that is, relative to the two other factors decision makers have to take into account:

1. 'local' circumstances; for example, it may not be possible to change an emergency service such that care is delivered by consultants due to the difficulties of recruiting and paying for the number of consultants required;
2. the political context in which the service is delivered; for example, the introduction of nurse practitioners may be opposed by the public, or the closure of a low-volume but much-loved local hospital service may be vigorously resisted by the community.

Resource constraints and political pressures do not, however, negate the need for evidence; on the contrary, the need for research-based knowledge is heightened even though these other factors may outweigh the scientific evidence when the final decision is taken.

Reference

1. McKIBBON, K.A. and WALKER, C.J. (1994) *Beyond ACP Journal Club: how to harness MEDLINE for therapy problems [Editorial]*. ACP Journal Club Jul-Aug; 121 Suppl 1: A10–2.

3.2 TESTS

'Gus and Wes had succeeded in elevating medicine to an exact science. All men reporting on sick call with temperatures above 102 were rushed to hospital. All those except Yossarian reporting on sick call with temperatures below 102 had their gums and toes painted with gentian violet solution and were given a laxative to throw away into the bushes. All those reporting on sick call with temperatures of exactly 102 were asked to return in an hour to have their temperatures taken again.'

Joseph Heller, *Catch 22*, 1962

3.2.1 Dimensions and definitions

A test may be defined as any measurement used to identify individuals who could benefit from therapeutic intervention. These measurements may be:

- the presence or absence of a symptom – something a patient feels;
- the presence or absence of a sign – something a clinician can detect;
- laboratory or radiological measurements.

The term 'test' is often used as a synonym for diagnostic test, but tests may have a function other than that of diagnosis:

- to monitor the effect of treatment and therefore to be used to determine whether treatment should be continued, changed or stopped;
- to provide information about prognosis (the future course of a disease);
- to indicate either the presence/absence of or the degree of risk.

Screening is discussed separately in Section 3.3 because the process involves more than the performance of a test: the beneficial effects of screening tests must be balanced against the adverse effects of any intervention resulting from those screening tests.

Some of the criteria used to assess the efficacy of tests are the same as those used to assess that of therapies, namely, effectiveness, safety, acceptability and cost. The criteria specific to the assessment of tests are:

- sensitivity;
- specificity;
- the relationship between sensitivity and specificity;
- predictive value and likelihood ratio.

3.2.1.1 Sensitivity and specificity

Diagnostic tests are used for many purposes, but at their simplest can be only positive or negative: people are shown either to have the disease or not to have the disease. However, few tests are perfect. Most people who do not have the disease will have a negative result (true negatives), but some people with negative test results may actually have the disease (false negatives). Most people who do have the disease will have a positive test result (true positives), but some people with positive test results will not have the disease (false positives). Thus, four types of test result may be obtained as a combination of these two variables (Fig. 3.2).

This balance between true positives and false positives and between true negatives and false negatives is expressed by two criteria which are used to judge all diagnostic tests:

- sensitivity;
- specificity.

Sensitivity is the proportion of people with the disease who are detected as having it by the test.
Specificity is the proportion of people without the disease who are correctly reassured by a negative test.

		Disease	
		Present	Absent
Test	Positive	True positive A	B False positive
	Negative	False negative C	D True negative

Fig. 3.2
The four types of test result

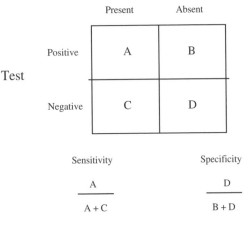

Fig. 3.3
Calculation of sensitivity and specificity of a diagnostic test

A method for calculating the sensitivity and specificity of a diagnostic test is shown in Fig. 3.3.

3.2.1.2 Sensitivity and positive predictive value

Sensitivity and specificity are constant criteria that can be applied to any diagnostic test irrespective of the characteristics of the population on which the test is used. However, the significance of a test result is determined not only by the sensitivity and the specificity of the test, but also by the prevalence of the condition in the population upon which the test is used.

The results of conducting a diagnostic test that has a 90% sensitivity and a 90% specificity in two different populations (both $n = 1000$), one in which there is a low prevalence of a disease and the other in which there is a high prevalence, are presented in Matrices 3.1 and 3.2. The results in Matrix 3.1 reflect the situation in hospital practice, in which 50% of the patients have the disease (high prevalence): as the test's sensitivity is 90%, 90% of the people who have a positive test result will have the disease and the test has a positive predictive value of 90%. The results in Matrix 3.2 reflect the situation in general practice in which only 10% of patients have the disease (low prevalence): even though the sensitivity is 90%, the positive predictive value is only 50%.

This difference in the predictive value of a test despite the constancy of sensitivity and specificity is the main reason that:

Test \ Disease	Present	Absent
Positive	450	50
Negative	50	450
Total	500	500

Matrix 3.1
Prevalence of disease 50%

Test \ Disease	Present	Absent
Positive	90	90
Negative	10	810
Total	100	900

Matrix 3.2
Prevalence of disease 10%

- hospital doctors believe GPs miss 'easy' diagnoses;
- GPs believe hospital doctors overinvestigate.

The criteria of sensitivity, specificity and predictive value are relevant for all tests whether numerical or perceptual.

1. Numerical tests

Some tests generate results in the form of numerical values, for example, biochemical tests. When test results are expressed numerically, the meaning of those results will vary depending upon whether the test has been used to identify:

- certain individuals within the range of a single population, for example, those who have raised blood pressure (Fig. 3.4);
- the presence of two populations, for example, those who do or do not have spina bifida, where the test results of each population will fall within a range of values that overlap with each other (Fig. 3.5).

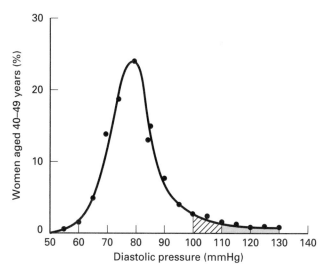

Fig. 3.4
Frequency distribution of diastolic pressure in females aged 40–49 years in a London population sample. The tinted area shows patients known to be at risk and known to benefit from treatment. The hatched area, comprising pressures of 100–110 mmHg, represents subjects who are also at risk but it is not yet known if they would benefit from hypotensive therapy. Subjects in the remaining white area are those with 'normal' blood pressures. (From Pickering, 1974, Hypertension: Courses, Consequences and Management, 2nd edition. Edinburgh, Churchill Livingstone, with permission.)

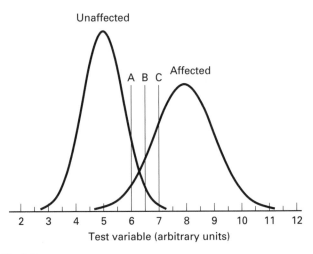

Unaffected

Affected

A B C

2 3 4 5 6 7 8 9 10 11 12

Test variable (arbitrary units)

Fig. 3.5
Hypothetical example of the detection rate and false-positive rate of a screening test at three different cut-off levels, A, B and C

From Fig. 3.4, it can be seen how different test values can be chosen to delineate those identified as having 'normal' blood pressure from those identified as having 'high' blood pressure. From Fig. 3.5, it can be seen how the cut-off point between positive and negative can be varied. The choice of any numerical cut-off point within a data set, whether applied to a single population or to two populations, is arbitrary. The choice of a cut-off point is difficult because there is always a trade-off between sensitivity and specificity (see Section 3.2.1.3).

2. Perceptual tests
Some tests, known as perceptual tests, are dependent upon the use of a human being as a measuring tool. Human perception is used to distinguish positive from negative, by:

• seeing, e.g. the analysis of X-rays or histopathological specimens;
• hearing, e.g. the detection of heart murmurs;
• palpation, e.g. the detection of congenital dislocation of the hip.

Any test that involves human perception and judgement is bedevilled by variability of reporting on results. There are two forms of variability.

1. Intraobserver variability is the phenomenon in which the same observer classifies the same test result differently on two separate occasions.
2. Interobserver variability is the phenomenon in which different observers classify the same test results differently.

Within epidemiology, the phenomenon of interobserver variability is widely accepted; it is also gaining acceptance within the profession. Indeed, this phenomenon should be recognised as an inevitable consequence of the use of perceptual tests. Unfortunately, within the legal system, interobserver variability is interpreted categorically as one observer being 'right' and another being 'wrong'.

3.2.1.3   Between a rock and a hard place

As any threshold is an arbitrarily selected value, it is possible to change the value of the threshold and therefore the balance between positive and negative results. At any particular threshold, the balance of false positives and false negatives will be different. This illustrates one of the central principles of testing, namely, that any increase in sensitivity is usually accompanied by a decrease in specificity and vice versa. The greater the degree to which a service is designed never to miss a diagnosis, that is, many measures have been taken to increase the sensitivity of the test(s) used, the greater will be the number of false-positive results generated. As sensitivity increases, a point is reached at which very small increases in sensitivity are accompanied by very large decreases in specificity, i.e. the number of false-positive results increases.

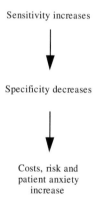

Sensitivity increases

Specificity decreases

Costs, risk and patient anxiety increase

An increase in the number of false-positive test results increases patient anxiety, the costs of treatment and the risk associated with unnecessary treatment.

The results of two studies published recently provide evidence of the disadvantage of increasing sensitivity. The sensitivity of magnetic resonance imaging (MRI) in the detection of pituitary adenoma (tumour) can be increased by the administration of certain chemicals to those undergoing imaging. In one study, the images from 100 healthy volunteers were mixed with those from 57 patients who had pituitary adenoma; the images were read by three experts independently. Ten per cent of the healthy volunteers were diagnosed as having adenoma, which is a very rare disease.[1] In another study, the MR images of 98 asymptomatic people were mixed with those of 27 people who had back pain;

the images were read by two experts independently. Sixty-four percent of the asymptomatic individuals were classified as 'abnormal'.[2] In the accompanying editorial,[3] it was stated that: 'The recent increase in the rates of lumbar spine surgery may be related in part to the availability of new imaging techniques'.

3.2.1.4 Tests: the producer's perspective

The number of new tests developed, particularly biochemical tests, is increasing each year, and the rate of increase will accelerate as new genetic tests become available.

Manufacturers rarely evaluate their tests using criteria such as sensitivity or predictive value. The manufacturer is usually satisfied if:

- the chemical specification of the test has been improved: for example, if proteins can be separated with increased precision;
- the performance of the test is easier and requires a lower level of skill from laboratory staff;
- the cost of the test has been reduced.

Those responsible for developing tests focus primarily on sensitivity, but this strategy carries a concomitant decrease in specificity (see Section 3.2.1.3).

For the decision maker in any health service, however, the perspective is different: although the manufacturers' criteria are relevant, criteria such as sensitivity are also important. Purchasers need to know whether a marginal increase in sensitivity leads to better outcomes for the population as a whole or for individual patients only.

3.2.1.5 Tests: the purchaser's perspective

To the developer of a test, increased test precision, for example, a narrower band on the spectroscope, is sufficient to justify the introduction of a new product; to the clinician, changes in sensitivity and specificity may provide sufficient justification. However, the purchaser responsible for the health of a population must take into account the impact that a new test, or an expansion of testing, has on the health of that population in terms not only of sensitivity but also of specificity and the number of false-positive diagnoses made. Any increase in the number of individuals having tests will result in an increase in the number of positive test results; some individuals with positive test results will have the disease, others will not (false positives) (see Fig. 3.6). However, even if the false positives are excluded and all the people who have a positive test actually have the disease, the effects of increasing the number of people tested may be simply to detect people with less severe disease (see Fig. 3.6).

Research conducted in the USA has demonstrated that an increase in the number of tests performed increases the volume of treatment. In a cohort study of 12 coronary angiography service areas in New England in which the intensity of investigation of individuals with chest pain varied,[4] a positive relationship was found between total stress test rates and the rates of subsequent coronary angiography; a strong relationship was also shown between coronary angiography and revascularisation. Furthermore, from an analysis of the Medicare National Claims History files which cover 30 million elderly Americans, it was found that investigation rates increased markedly over a 7-year period from 50% to 300%;[5] these increases in the rates of diagnostic testing were associated with an increase in the rates of administration of relevant procedures (see Table 3.2). It could be that the increased rate of testing revealed exactly the same type of cases as had been diagnosed previously, but this assumption cannot be made immediately.

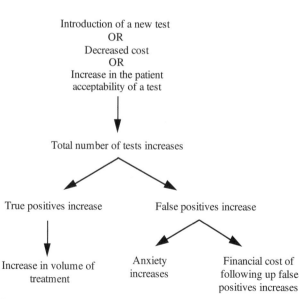

Fig. 3.6

Table 3.2 (Source: Verrilli and Welch[5])

Investigation	Treatment
Cardiac catheterisation	Cardiac revascularisation (CABG and PTCA)
Spinal imaging (CT and MRI)	Back surgery
Swallowing studies	Percutaneous gastrostomy
Mammography	Breast biopsy and excision
Prostate biopsy	Prostatectomy

The benefits obtained from increased expenditure on testing may decline as the volume of testing increases; however, these observational studies were not of a sufficiently sensitive design to address such issues. It is clear, however, that increased diagnostic testing is one of the major factors leading to an increase in the volume of treatment. Any attempt to control the volume of treatment that does not include the control of the development of diagnostic services is doomed to failure.

3.2.2 Searching

Good advice on searching for evidence about tests is given in the *ACP Journal Club*.[6]

A MEDLINE search has five components (see Table 3.3).

Table 3.3 Components of a MEDLINE search for a test

Component	Example
The clinical problem	Coeliac disease
The test	Gliadin antibody test
The characteristics of the test	Sensitivity and specificity
Study design	Review
The time frame	1985–1995

In terms of study design, the first step is to look for meta-analysis of studies using:

- the term 'meta-analysis';
- text word 'meta';
- any word starting with 'analy'.

In addition to text words, MeSH headings can be used when searching for papers on tests. The relevant MeSH headings are:

- sensitivity and specificity;
- predictive value of tests;
- false-negative reactions;
- false-positive reactions;
- diagnosis, differential;
- diagnostic test;
- diagnostic service;
- routine diagnostic test;
- diagnosis.

If you wish to limit the number of MeSH headings, use:

- sensitivity;
- diagnosis (NB: 'explode' the term 'diagnosis' if asked).

3.2.3 Appraisal

Appraisal is a two-stage procedure.

1. What is the best method for appraising a test?
2. How good is any of the research found?

The best method for appraising a test is a large well-designed RCT that has patient outcomes, such as survival or quality of life, as end-points. Unfortunately, RCTs of tests are scarce. As a compromise, it is probably necessary to accept results from research studies designed to have better test performance as an end-point, for example, greater sensitivity of a test for a disease for which it has been shown in an RCT that intervention is effective.

As large trials are rarely feasible, it is essential to find reviews of small studies in which meta-analysis of the data from the individual studies has been undertaken irrespective of whether the test results are presented as dichotomous (i.e. 'positive' or 'negative') or continuous. Irwig et al[7] have developed Guidelines for Meta-analyses Evaluating Diagnostic Tests; their checklist for evaluating meta-analyses of diagnostic tests is shown in Box 3.1, which can be used to supplement the general guidance on appraising systematic reviews (see Section 5.2.3).

Box 3.1 Checklist for evaluating meta-analyses of diagnostic tests (Source: Irwig et al[7])

- Is there a clear statement about:
  - the test of interest?
  - the disease of interest and the reference standard by which it is measured?
  - the clinical question and context?
- Is the objective to evaluate a single test or to compare the accuracy of different tests?
- Is the literature retrieval procedure described with search and link terms given?
- Are inclusion and exclusion criteria stated?
- Are studies assessed by two or more readers?
  - Do the authors explain how disagreements between readers were resolved?
- Is a full listing of diagnostic accuracy and study characteristics given for each primary study?
- Does the method of pooling sensitivity and specificity take account of their interdependence?
- When multiple test categories are available, are they used in the summary?
- Is the relation examined between estimates of diagnostic accuracy and study validity of the primary studies for each of the following design characteristics:
  - appropriate reference standard?
  - independent assessment of the test or tests and reference standard?
- In comparative studies, were all of the tests of interest applied to each patient or were patients randomly allocated to the tests?
- Are analytic methods used that estimated whether study design flaws affect diagnostic accuracy rather than just test threshold?
- Is the relation examined between estimates of diagnostic accuracy and characteristics of the patients and test?
- Are analytic methods used which differentiate whether characteristics affect diagnostic accuracy or test threshold?

If there are no meta-analyses available, individual studies must be appraised. For this type of appraisal the McMaster checklist can be used (see Box 3.2).

3.2.4 Getting research into practice

It is rarely necessary to promote the use of new tests of proven effectiveness for two reasons:

1. there is so little proof of effectiveness available;
2. there are no controls to restrict the introduction of new tests.

In fact, new tests, particularly biochemical tests, flood into practice. The main challenge, therefore, is stopping starting, that is, controlling the introduction of new tests (see Section 7.3.4.2).

Box 3.2 Methodological questions for appraising journal articles about diagnostic tests (Source: McMaster University[8])

The best articles evaluating diagnostic tests will meet most or all of the following eight criteria.

1. Was there an independent, 'blind' comparison with a 'gold standard' of diagnosis?
2. Was the setting for the study, as well as the filter through which study patients passed, adequately described?
3. Did the patient sample include an appropriate spectrum of mild and severe, treated and untreated disease, plus individuals with different but commonly confused disorders?
4. Were the tactics for carrying out the test described in sufficient detail to permit their exact replication?
5. Was the reproducibility of the test (precision) and its interpretation (observer variation) determined?
6. Was the term 'normal' defined sensibly? (Gaussian, percentile, risk factor, culturally desirable, diagnostic or therapeutic?)
7. If the test is advocated as part of a cluster or sequence of tests, was its contribution to the overall validity of the cluster or sequence determined?
8. Was the 'utility' of the test determined? (Were patients really better off for it?)

References

1. HALL, W.A., LUCIANO, M.G., DOPPMAN, J.L. et al. (1994) *Pituitary magnetic resonance imaging in normal human volunteers: occult adenomas in the general population*. Ann. Intern. Med. 120: 817–20.
2. JENSEN, M.C., BRANT-ZAWADKI, M.N., OBUCHOWSKI, N. et al. (1994) *Magnetic resonance imaging of the lumbar spine in people without back pain*. New Eng. J. Med. 331: 69–73.
3. *Magnetic resonance imaging of the lumbar spine. Terrific test or tar baby?* [Editorial]. New Eng. J. Med. 331: 115–16.
4. WENNBERG, D.E., KELLETT, M.A., DICKENS, J.D. Jr. et al. (1996) *The association between local diagnostic testing intensity and invasive cardiac procedures*. JAMA 275: 1161–4.
5. VERRILLI, D. and WELCH, H.G. (1996) *The impact of diagnostic testing on therapeutic interventions*. JAMA 275: 1189–91.
6. McKIBBON, K.A. and WALKER-DILKS, C.J. (1994) *Beyond ACP Journal Club: how to harness MEDLINE for diagnostic problems [Editorial]*. ACP Journal Club Sept-Oct; 121 Suppl 2: A10–2.
7. IRWIG, L., TOSTESON, A.N.A., GATSONIS, C. et al. (1994) *Guidelines for meta-analyses evaluating diagnostic tests*. Ann. Intern. Med. 120: 667–76.
8. McMASTER UNIVERSITY *Critical Appraisal Card from Department of Clinical Epidemiology and Biostatistics*. McMaster University, Hamilton, Ontario, Canada.

3.3 SCREENING

> **'Screen**: an apparatus used in the sifting of grain, coal, etc. 1573.'
>
> *Shorter Oxford English Dictionary*

Dear Reader,

Empathise with Jock Armstrong and Will Taggart. They glared at one another across the row of straw which had been spewed forth from the Claas combine harvester, a massive mechanical monument, now still in the blackening wheat of a Scottish harvest field.

'Look at the wheat on the ground, man, 'roared Jock, 'You've set the holes in the screen too big so that you could hash on for the next job.'

'Ach, away man,' growled Will, his eyes shining forth in a face almost black with stour.

'I'm due at Balanin the night and she's blocked solid with chaff because the screen's set as small as they'll go.'

The peewit cried in the Galloway sky, its whooping call like a referee's whistle keeping the two opposing forces on either side of the line of straw: the farmer wanting the screen set so that not a single grain falls to earth; the contractor knowing that the smaller the holes, the more often will chaff, grain, stones and straw build up and cause first colic then complete obstruction in his combine harvester. And with him wanting to drive as fast as he can to the next farm to combine barley before the rain curtails harvesting (and income).

Commentary

Farmer or contractor; saving of grain or saving of time; sensitivity or specificity – the eternal tensions in any screening programme.

3.3.1 Dimensions and definitions

In a screening programme, a test, or a series of tests, is performed on a population that has neither the signs nor the symptoms of the disease being sought but whose members have some characteristic that identifies them as being at risk from that disease, the outcome of which can be improved by early detection and treatment.

Screening may be organised proactively, by inviting members of the population at risk to attend for testing, as is the case in breast cancer screening, or opportunistically, for example, blood pressure monitoring performed during the course of a patient's visit to their general practitioner about another possibly unrelated health problem. The evaluation is the same for both types of programme management.

In contrast, case finding is a process of identifying individuals who are asymptomatic but who are at risk of disease because they are related to a symptomatic individual: for example, contacting all the first-degree relatives of an individual who has had a myocardial infarction at the age of 42 years and who has been diagnosed as having familial hypercholesterolaemia.

When screening is discussed, the term is usually taken to refer to a single test, for example, mammography within the breast cancer screening programme. However, screening actually consists of all the steps in a programme from the identification of the population at risk to the diagnosis of the disease or its precursor in certain individuals to the treatment of those individuals. In the case of breast cancer screening, the steps range from the identification of women over 50 years old (the group that will benefit) to the accurate histopathological diagnosis and effective treatment of breast cancer.

Thus, the effectiveness of any screening programme is determined by:

- the sensitivity of the series of tests applied to the population;
- the effectiveness of the therapy offered to those individuals discovered to have the condition.

> Screening effectiveness
> =
> test accuracy + therapeutic effectiveness

It is the involvement of a subset of the entire population that distinguishes screening from clinical practice. In clinical practice, a person concerned about a health problem seeks help knowing that not every patient benefits and some people experience side-effects; in screening, healthy individuals are drawn into a health service, only a small proportion of whom will benefit and those diagnosed as false positives will suffer harm, having previously been well. Thus, the balance of good to harm is of particular importance in decisions about screening.

3.3.1.1 The changing balance of good and harm

Screening programmes, like any other intervention, have the potential to do both good and harm. However, the balance between good and harm will change with the frequency of testing and the quality of the programme. Cervical screening at a frequency of once every 3 years probably results in an increase of only 7% in effectiveness when compared with an effectiveness of 84% claimed for cervical screening every 5 years. The beneficial effects of screening illustrate the law of diminishing returns (Fig. 3.7A) whereas the adverse effects of screening, or of any other intervention, usually follow a straight line (Fig. 3.7B). The greater the number of individuals involved in a screening programme, the greater will be the number experiencing side-effects (Fig. 3.7C). Thus, the ratio of benefits to harm changes as the number of individuals screened increases.

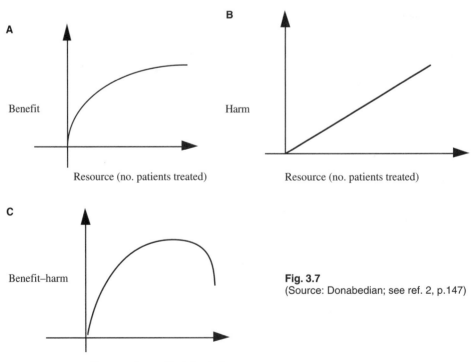

Fig. 3.7
(Source: Donabedian; see ref. 2, p.147)

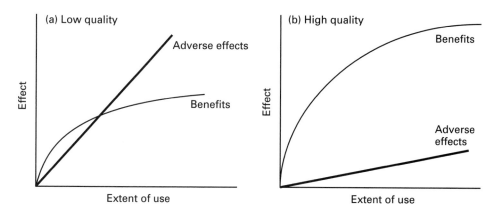

Fig. 3.8
Benefits and adverse effects of low- and high-quality screening

If the quality of the screening programme is low, the benefits are reduced and adverse effects increase (Fig. 3.8); if an adequate level of quality is not achieved, there may be a point at which the harm done by screening is greater than the good. Thus, the decision to introduce screening must be taken with the greatest of care.

3.3.2 Searching

A MEDLINE search has five useful components (see Table 3.4).

Table 3.4 Components of a MEDLINE search for a screening programme

Component	Example
The health problem	Breast cancer
The principal test	Mammography
The type of intervention	Screening
Study design	Review or RCT
The time frame	1985–1995

3.3.3 Appraisal

The first step in appraisal is to identify the research design most likely to be helpful. In screening, it is the RCT or a systematic review of RCTs.

Proponents of the introduction of any screening programme sometimes base their argument on cohort studies, which are designed to follow a series of people who have had a screening test and compare their survival with that of the general population. However, this is a poor method of evaluating screening, principally because of what is called lead-time bias.

Imagine a disease that has a natural history of 10 years from its beginning to its fatal end, and that causes symptoms after 5 years, which usually prompt the sufferer to visit a doctor; the survival time from the point of symptomatic diagnosis is five years (Fig. 3.9A). A test that enables a diagnosis to be made at an earlier, presymptomatic stage, for example at 3 years, will apparently increase survival time (Fig. 3.9B). This apparent increase in survival time does not necessarily mean that screening is effective; it may simply mean that the person with the presymptomatic disease found by screening is aware of the condition for 7 years as opposed to 5 – this is referred to as lead-time bias. It is essential that any screening programme is evaluated within an RCT which has been designed with death as the outcome in order to control for lead-time bias.

The classic set of criteria for appraising screening tests were developed by Wilson and Jungner[1] in 1968 (see Box 3.3). Although these criteria have been useful, they are weak in the following ways.

- There is insufficient emphasis on the adverse effects of screening and the need to ensure that a programme does more good than harm. Although these factors were important in the 1960s, in the context of a better informed, more assertive public, which is more likely to sue if harm is done, it is essential to concentrate on these factors.
- The criteria state that an 'accepted treatment' should be available, but many accepted treatments are either ineffective or of unproven efficacy.
- There is no discussion of the quality of the evidence upon which the decision should be made.

A more suitable set of criteria for current use has been developed (see Box 3.4).

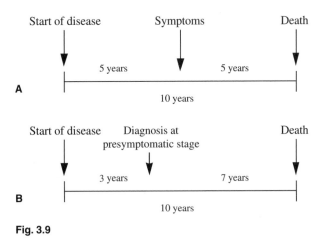

Fig. 3.9

Box 3.3 Criteria for appraising screening developed in the 1960s (Source: Wilson and Jungner[1])

- The condition sought should be an important health problem.
- There should be an accepted treatment for patients with recognized disease.
- Facilities for diagnosis and treatment should be available.
- There should be a recognizable latent or early symptomatic stage.
- There should be a suitable test or examination.
- The test should be acceptable to the population.
- The natural history of the condition, including development from latent to declared disease, should be adequately understood.
- There should be an agreed policy on whom to treat as patients.
- The cost of case-finding (including diagnosis and treatment of patients diagnosed) should be economically balanced in relation to possible expenditure on medical care as a whole.
- Case-finding should be a continuing process and not a 'once and for all' project.

Box 3.4 1990s criteria for appraising screening

Is there evidence from a good-quality RCT (see Section 5.3), analysed on an intention-to-treat basis, that the proposed screening programme is effective in reducing mortality?

If the answer is 'no', there is 'no' case for implementation. If 'yes', the following questions should be addressed.

- How many people have to be screened to find one case or prevent one death (the number needed to treat [NNT], see Section 6.3.3.1)?
- How many people would be adversely affected by screening:
  – per thousand screened?
  – per life saved?
- How broad are the confidence intervals around the estimated size of the beneficial effect and what are, at each end of the confidence intervals, the:
  – NNT?
  – numbers adversely affected?
  (This question is particularly important because the size of the effect found in the ideal circumstances of the trial may not be reproducible in a routine screening service.)
- What are the financial costs of the screening programme and what health benefits would be obtained by using those resources allocated to screening on:
  a) other ways of managing the health problem the screening programme has been designed to tackle, for example, improving the treatment of breast cancer?
  b) other services for that population the screening programme is designed to benefit?
  c) any other service for any other population group?

3.3.4   Getting research into practice

Getting research into practice in a screening programme is a major undertaking, perhaps more so than for any other type of healthcare intervention. This is because the introduction of a new screening programme requires the concomitant introduction of a wide range of clinical interventions, together with management and information support systems that will enable quality to be assured. There must be:

- explicit agreed standards of good practice;
- an information system that enables performance against those standards to be measured;
- the authority to take action if standards are not achieved.

For a screening programme to do more good than harm requires not simply the demonstration that it is possible to achieve this in a research setting, but also an emphasis on quality in practice that will allow the potential to be realised in any setting.

3.3.5   Aphoristic warnings

The decision to introduce screening is relatively easy; resolving the problems that may result from it can be much more difficult. For this reason, some aphorisms on screening are provided for the reader to ponder before succumbing to the temptations of screening.

> A stitch in time does not necessarily save nine.
>
> The decision to introduce a new screening programme should be taken as carefully as the decision to build a new hospital.
>
> Never think about screening tests, only about screening programmes.
>
> Screening programmes shown to be efficacious in a research setting require an obsession with quality to be effective in a service setting.
>
> The public are overoptimistic about screening; professionals are overpessimistic.
>
> Finding 'asymptomatic' disease by means of screening always increases the length of time a person knows s/he has the disease; this increased period of awareness should not be confused with increased survival.

All screening programmes do harm; some can do good as well.

The harm from a screening programme starts immediately; the good takes longer to appear. Therefore, the first effect of any programme, even an effective one, is to impair the health of the population.

A screening programme without false positives will miss too many cases to be effective.

Like the tightrope walker above Niagara Falls, any screening programme must balance false negatives and false positives.

A screening programme without false negatives will cause unnecessary harm to the healthy population.

For the distressed patient seeking help, the clinician does what s/he can; for the healthy person recruited to screening, only the best possible service will suffice.

Screening programmes should be run with firm management. If quality falls, a screening programme that was doing more good than harm may then do more harm than good.

Though insignificant to the population, a single false positive can be of devastating significance to the individual.

If a screening programme is not supported by a quality assurance system, it should be stopped. Quality assurance encompasses the essentials: standards, information and authority to act.

If a quality assurance programme is not generating at least one major public enquiry every 3 years, it is ineffective.

At best, screening is a zero gratitude business.

Reference

1. WILSON, J.M.G. and JUNGNER, G. (1968) *Principles and Practice of Screening for Disease*. World Health Organization, Geneva.

3.4 HEALTH POLICY AND MANAGEMENT CHANGES

3.4.1 Dimensions and definitions

Before discussing health policy in detail it is important to propose a working definition that distinguishes policy from management. Changes in policy may be for one of two reasons:

1. to improve health;
2. to change the way in which health services are funded and held accountable.

The objectives within healthcare policy changes might include:

- to delegate responsibility for decision making about the use of resources;
- to increase the number of people involved in decisions about resources;
- to increase incentives to achieve better value for money;
- to clarify and strengthen accountability;
- to improve performance against targets (for instance, Health of the Nation targets in the UK);
- to change the way in which money for healthcare is raised, for example, by introducing or increasing charges;
- to improve patient care.

Although such changes are often political, that is, decided upon by politicians, they always have managerial consequences.

Managers can also introduce changes, either to increase efficiency and quality or to ensure that policy objectives are met using the resources available, but such changes have only indirect effects on clinical decision making. The overall objectives of these managerial changes are to improve:

- efficiency;
- quality;
- accountability;
- acceptability.

For example, managers may:

- introduce schemes of quality improvement;
- increase investment in training;
- change managerial structures either to increase professional involvement or to decrease the amount of time wasted by professionals in management, or both;

- change the financial computing system;
- introduce measures to involve patients in the process of care;
- externalise services, such as cleaning or pathology.

However, politicians do make policy decisions that affect clinical practice directly. One such decision has been to influence GP prescribing habits by excluding certain drugs from the list from which doctors can choose; another such decision has been the introduction of case management (a US term) or care management (a UK term) to improve the quality of care for severely mentally ill people.

In classifying health policy, the usual approach is to use the determinants of health:

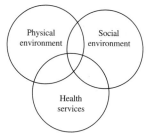

- the physical environment;
- the social environment;
- health services.

Changes in the physical and social environments are the main factors influencing:

- the incidence of disease;
- the number of new cases of a disease in the population.

These factors also influence the prevalence of the disease in the number of people with the disease.

With effective health services, it is possible to prevent or reduce the prevalence of disease (by curing it) or to alleviate its burden by minimising the disability that disease causes.

Policies that have as a primary focus changes in the physical or social environment are health policies, sometimes called public health policies; those that have health service funding, organisation or accountability as a focus are conventionally known as healthcare policies.

3.4.2 Searching

For healthcare policy, there may be evidence from RCTs, such as the one that failed to demonstrate a beneficial effect of case management in people who had severe mental illness.[1,2] For policies such as those that influence the finance and organisation of a health service, descriptive studies of other comparable health services provide the evidence most easily available.

For health or public health policies, the evidence may be available within more conventional scientific forms:

- the case-control study (Section 5.4);
- the cohort study (Section 5.5);
- cluster analysis (Section 7.5.3).

It may be productive to search HealthSTAR, a specialist database (see Appendix I).

3.4.3 Appraisal

It is a common belief that work on health policy or health service management is difficult to translate from one country to another because of the myriad social, cultural and political differences. Although it is true it is often not possible to transfer a policy or managerial option directly from one country to another, research on health policy and management in different countries can be illuminating.

If the healthcare system in operation is similar, any managerial initiatives are of interest; if the healthcare system is different, then it can be regarded as if a 'natural' experiment were taking place. In a 'natural' experiment, different approaches to the same problem can be compared despite the fact that those different approaches were not planned in a research setting but arose by reason of different circumstances.

Even when the social, cultural and political circumstances of a country are very different to those of one's own there is much to be learned. Anthropological studies, such as that by Frankel described in *The Huli Response to Illness*,[3] can provide many insights into the human response to disease, illness and treatment which may be helpful to policy makers and managers. Indeed, managers and policy makers may have underestimated the potential for learning from research conducted in other countries and within different cultures.

A checklist of useful questions for the appraisal of research on policy is shown in Box 3.5.

Box 3.5

- Was a clear hypothesis set out?
- If the study was designed to investigate the effect of some intervention or change, were the data gathered before and after the introduction of the intervention/change comparable?
- Were other confounding variables taken into account when the conclusions were drawn?
- Did the explanations given accord with the data presented?

3.4.4 Getting research into practice

As individuals usually have strong views about what is right in terms of policy or management, there may be greater resistance to implementing knowledge derived from research than that encountered when promoting the adoption of research findings in clinical practice. If a policy is based primarily on an ideology, or if a management change stems from the personal conviction of an individual manager, then evidence that such a policy or management change is ineffective or counterproductive is likely to meet with dogged resistance. A policy maker may be defensive about challenges to his/her ideology and the manager may regard any challenges as a personal affront. It is important, however, that a double standard is not introduced, namely, that policy makers and managers do not exhort clinicians to implement research findings in clinical practice when they themselves are either not actively searching for evidence or failing to implement knowledge derived from research when it is presented to them.

References

1. MARSHALL, M. (1996) *Case management: a dubious practice [Editorial].* Br. Med. J. 312: 523–4.
2. MARSHALL, M., GRAY, A., LOCKWOOD, A. and GREEN, R. (1996) *Case management for people with severe mental disorders.* In: Adams, C., Anderson, J., De Jesus Mari, J. (eds) *Schizophrenia Module of The Cochrane Database of Systematic Reviews [Updated 27 February 1996].* The Cochrane Collaboration; Issue 3. Update Software, Oxford.
3. FRANKEL, S. (1986) *The Huli Response to Illness.* Cambridge University Press, Cambridge.

PROLOGUE 4

Dear Reader,

Empathise with Jair de Jesus Mari, Professor of Psychiatry in São Paulo. September is hot in São Paulo, sometimes oppressively so. However, it was not the heat that bothered Jair in 1994. He was frustrated with the process of publishing scientific literature. For more than a year, he had laboured to summarise all the trials of psychosocial family interventions in schizophrenia that could be found by hand searching psychiatric journals. His review, based on six trials, was submitted to a prestigious journal in August 1993; it was published in August 1994[1] after a delay that was torment to him. He had received praise from colleagues and felt satisfied when he finally saw his review in print. One month later it was out of date; two further trials, both from China, had been published in another journal. He swore: the equivalent of 'bloody hell' in Portuguese. What should he do now? Write a letter to the first journal, perhaps, but he wanted to revise the meta-analysis and base the revision on all eight trials. Anyway, those who read the letter would not necessarily have the original article to hand when they read it; what's more, letters are not peer reviewed so they are not necessarily taken seriously by readers. Jair de Jesus Mari faced an insoluble dilemma.

Commentary

Jair's dilemma cannot be solved on paper, but it is possible to resolve electronically.

All decision makers should have computer access to the best information about the effectiveness of any intervention, that being a systematic review of trials based on a complete search of the literature, which also:

- *can be quickly updated when new evidence appears;*
- *has summaries of the original trials available;*
- *can be used by decision makers because practical implications, as well as scientific conclusions, are highlighted;*
- *has a responsive 'letters' column, such that all comments/criticisms and the author's replies are available instantaneously.*

The Cochrane Library, which is available on compact disk, now provides such a facility; the review by Mari and Streiner[2] meets all of the above criteria.

References

1. MARI, J.J. and STREINER, D. (1994) *An overview of family interventions and relapse in schizophrenia.* Psychol. Med. 23: 565–78.
2. MARI, J.J. and STREINER, D. (1996) *Family intervention for those with schizophrenia.* In: Adams, C., Anderson, J. and De Jesus Mari, J. (eds) *Schizophrenia Module of The Cochrane Database of Systematic Reviews, 1996 [Updated 27 February 1996].* The Cochrane Collaboration, Issue 3. Update Software, Oxford.

CHAPTER 4

SEARCHING FOR EVIDENCE

4.1 THE SEARCHER'S PROBLEMS

1. Absence of high-quality evidence

There is only a small amount of high-quality evidence available on which to base a decision, unless the decision is about cardiac services. The legacy of years of research is that the available evidence is not best suited to the needs of healthcare decision makers. This is illustrated by the data presented in Table 4.1; it can be seen that there are relatively few papers written about common conditions whereas there are numerous papers about relatively uncommon conditions. However, this fact should not be used as a reason to challenge investigator-driven research. To take a case in point, the papers on slow virus diseases of the central nervous system (CNS) may now be of greater

Table 4.1 The index of interest in various diagnoses (number of papers listed in Index Medicus 1986 in English/discharges and deaths (D&D) from hospital in-patient enquiry × 1000) (Source: Frankel and West[1])

Diagnoses	Discharges and deaths	Index of interest (Papers/D&D x 1000)
Slow virus diseases of CNS	40	2000
Myasthenia gravis	930	156
Crohn's disease	6670	44
Carcinoma of the breast	41 220	33
Rheumatoid arthritis	26 060	27
Carcinoma of the bronchus	54 440	20
Myocardial infarction	102 720	10
Cerebrovascular disease	111 250	7.7
Irritable bowel syndrome, etc.*	19 840	6.7
Cataract	54 990	6.5
Hip replacement	37 400	5.0
Haemorrhoids	20 700	1.0
Inguinal hernia	64 400	0.8
Tonsils and adenoids	76 600	0.7
Varicose veins	47 160	0.6

* Includes irritable bowel syndrome, dumping syndrome, constipation and other functional bowel disease.

relevance to decision makers considering the explosion of interest in bovine spongiform encephalopathy (BSE).

In the UK, one of the main functions of the NHS R&D Programme is the identification of NHS requirements for research-based knowledge (Fig. 4.1). The intention is to narrow the 'relevance gap' (see Fig. 4.1) and correct the

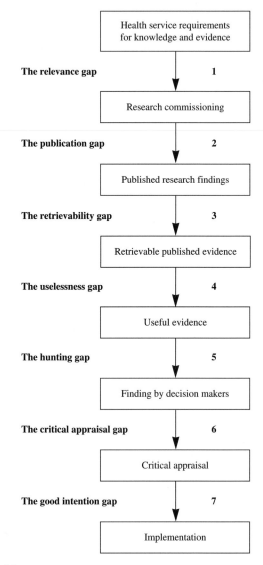

Fig. 4.1
The evidence gaps

imbalance; at present, however, many healthcare decisions must be made for which there is no high-quality evidence.

The Cochrane Database of Systematic Reviews (CDSR) (see Appendix I) is an electronic information source produced by the Cochrane Collaboration, the work of which will close the 'retrievability', 'uselessness', 'hunting' and 'critical appraisal' gaps also shown in Fig. 4.1.

The searcher's solution: The absence of excellent evidence does not make evidence-based decision making impossible; in this situation, what is required is the *best evidence available,* not the best evidence possible, using the classification shown in Table 4.2.

Table 4.2   The five strengths of evidence

Type	Strength of evidence
I	Strong evidence from at least one systematic review of multiple well-designed randomised controlled trials
II	Strong evidence from at least one properly designed randomised controlled trial of appropriate size
III	Evidence from well-designed trials without randomisation, single group pre-post, cohort, time series or matched case-control studies
IV	Evidence from well-designed non-experimental studies from more than one centre or research group
V	Opinions of respected authorities, based on clinical evidence, descriptive studies or reports of expert committees

2. *Unpublished evidence*

Any searcher must find the sources of evidence. Although much is made of the 'grey literature', that is, results of studies not published in scientific journals, the main source of evidence is the published literature. However, this is incomplete for three reasons:

- the 'sloppy' researcher – too many researchers fail to write up and submit their findings for publication;
- the 'coy' pharmaceutical company – nervous of revealing results that may not show the company's products in the most advantageous light;
- the 'biased' editor – keener to publish positive than negative results.[2]

The searcher's solution: It is appropriate to search for unpublished data if one is doing research, but if one is a busy decision maker it is not an effective use of time.

3. The limitations of electronic databases

There are many electronic databases, but the two principal sources are MEDLINE and EMBASE (see Appendix I). However, they cover only about 6000 of the 20 000 journals published worldwide and that coverage is primarily of English language journals.

The searcher's solution: The use of specialist databases (Appendix I) can minimise but not resolve the problems posed by the limitations of electronic databases. Access to The Cochrane Library diminishes the problems of searching for RCTs.

4. Inadequate indexing

Owing to inadequacies in the indexing of research papers, not only within journals but also within the electronic databases, many papers cannot be found. In general, only about half of the trials in MEDLINE can be found by even the best electronic searcher[3] (see Table 4.3).

Table 4.3 The findability gaps

	Experienced clinical searching	Skills gap	Optimal skilled MEDLINE searching	Indexing gap	Hand searching
% of RCTs found	18		52		94

One of the objectives of the Cochrane Collaboration is to make the results of more trials available to searchers. This objective is fulfilled by the hand searching of journals and the incorporation of any trials found into MEDLINE. Hand searching of the *British Medical Journal* and *Lancet* added greatly to the number of trials available on MEDLINE (Fig. 4.2).[4]

The searcher's solution: The use of good search strategies will minimise the impact of inadequate searching (see Appendix II). The best strategy is to have an expert searcher on hand but often one has to cope alone (see Section 4.3).

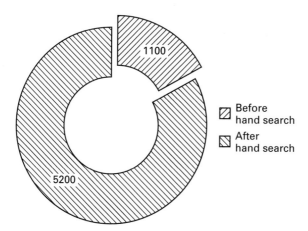

Fig. 4.2
British Medical Journal and The Lancet trials (1996–1994) identifiable in MEDLINE before and after the hand search (Source: McDonald et al[4], with permission, BMJ Publishing Group)

5. Misleading abstracts

A search produces papers. The quality of any search is measured by two criteria:

- accuracy: the proportion of findable articles that are found;
- precision: the proportion of articles found that are useful; the rest are 'junk'.

> Precision = 1 – 'junk'

Having found the articles, the next step is to identify and discard the 'junk'. Good searching increases accuracy but almost always decreases precision, i.e. it also uncovers 'junk'. The simplest way to identify 'junk' is to read the abstract, but it should be borne in mind that abstracts are written with a bias towards highlighting the most positive aspects of a paper.[5]

The searcher's solution: There are two guidelines for reading abstracts.

- If the abstract is unstructured, be suspicious.[6]
- If the abstract highlights negative findings, it may not be biased, but if it highlights positive findings appraise the methods section before accepting the paper as good-quality evidence.

6. Human frailty

Even when evidence is available and the articles are findable, an experienced clinical searcher may not discover them. In one study it was shown that, in addition to the problems of inadequate indexing which meant that only about half the trials were findable by the most skilled searcher, the experienced clinical searcher, despite having made frequent use of MEDLINE, found only half of the papers the expert found.[3]

The searcher's solution: Improve searching skills (see Sections 4.3.2 and 8.1).

References

1. FRANKEL, S. and WEST, R. (1993) *Rationing and rationality in the National Health Service.* Macmillan, Basingstoke, p 11.
2. EASTERBROOK, P.J., BERLIN, J.A., GOPALAN, R. and MATTHEWS, D.R. (1991) *Publication bias in clinical research.* Lancet 337: 867–72.
3. ADAMS, C.E., POWER, A., FREDERICK, K. and LEFEBVRE, C. (1994) *An investigation of the adequacy of MEDLINE searches for randomized controlled trials (RCTs) of the effects of mental health care.* Psychol. Med. 24: 741–8.
4. McDONALD, S.J., LEFEBVRE, C. and CLARKE, M.J. (1996) *Identifying reports of controlled trials in the BMJ and The Lancet.* Br. Med. J. 313: 1116-7.
5. GØTZSCHE, P. (1989) *Methodology and overt and hidden bias in reports of 196 double-blind trials of nonsteroidal anti-inflammatory drugs in rheumatoid arthritis.* Controlled Clinical Trials 10: 31–56.
6. AD HOC WORKING GROUP FOR CRITICAL APPRAISAL OF THE MEDICAL LITERATURE. (1987) *A proposal for more informative abstracts of clinical articles.* Ann. Intern. Med. 106: 598–604.

4.2   THE INFORMATION BROKER

The traditional role of the librarian is changing. As the next century approaches, the librarian will become an information broker, facilitating the interchange between those who need and those who provide information. The 'library' will also be different: not simply a room full stacks and shelves, but an information or evidence centre, linked to the world through the Web (see Section 7.1.4.1).

4.3   COPING ALONE

In managing the acquisition of knowledge there are two principal modes: proactive and reactive. A proactive style of knowledge management is to scan the literature regularly and thereby search for potentially relevant knowledge (predominantly a scanning activity). A reactive style of knowledge management is based on the principle that no decision maker will ever be able to anticipate all the questions that are likely to arise and therefore it is more effective to develop good searching skills and use them as and when required (predominantly a searching activity). Each decision maker must strike a balance between the two types of activities and define a mode of knowledge management most appropriate to needs and circumstances.

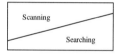

'Knowledge management'

Scanning

Searching

Pro-active   Reactive

4.3.1   Becoming a better scanner

When preparing a scanning strategy, use the checklist of questions shown in Box 4.1.

Box 4.1   Useful prompts in the preparation of a scanning strategy

- How many hours each week do I want to spend scanning for new knowledge?
- What sources of knowledge do I want to scan regularly?
- What sources of information will I not even open or look at?
- How can I ensure I miss nothing really important using this strategy?
- What checklists can I use to ensure I stick to my scanning objectives? (A Filofax weekly checklist is useful.)
- Is there anyone else who could develop, or already has developed, a scanning strategy with whom I could share the load?
- How can I review the benefits and weaknesses of this strategy at the end of the year?

4.3.2 Becoming a better searcher

There are two steps that can be taken to improve searching skills (see also Section 8.1).

1. Undertake formal training; ask the librarian if there are any searching training courses available.
2. Elicit the support of a librarian; first enrol for an induction session, then search with the librarian, and finally ask the librarian to review some searches completed without support to obtain feedback on sensitivity and precision.

4.3.3 Becoming better at critical appraisal

Formal training in critical appraisal is becoming increasingly available (see Section 8.2). If there is no access to formal training, take the following steps.

- Collect all the articles on critical appraisal listed in Appendix IIIA.
- Download the information from the book's Web site: http://www.ihs.ox.ac.uk/ebh.html
- Set up a problem-based journal club in order to work with colleagues to find and appraise articles relating to decisions that have to be made.

4.3.4 Becoming a better storekeeper

Information can be stored in many ways, but the most appropriate storing strategy is to use reference management software and store the articles on it using keywords (see Section 8.3). The paper copies can be filed alphabetically by first author.

4.3.5 Use it or lose it

Any decision makers within a health service who find, appraise and use evidence will contribute to changing the culture of the organisation in which they work (see Section 7.1). This course of action provides an example to other people who will discuss the evidence found and begin to find evidence themselves. As such, the skills of finding, appraising and storing evidence will be strengthened, not only within individuals but also throughout the organisation.

Further reading

HAYNES, R.B. (1995) *Current awareness and current access: ACP Journal Club goes electronic.* ACP Journal Club Jul–Aug; 123(1): A14.

McKIBBON, K.A. et al. (1995) *Beyond ACP Journal Club: how to harness MEDLINE for prognosis problems.* ACP Journal Club Jul–Aug; 123(1): A12–4.

PROLOGUE 5

Dear Reader,

Empathise with the epidemiologist. He stood in the dock, cool, calm and collected. The judge entered, adjusted her robes, peered over her half-moon spectacles, and imposed, by all the non-verbal signals commonly used in that particular form of theatre, her presence on the court.

'How do you plead?' she said, 'Guilty or not guilty?'

The epidemiologist replied, 'How will I know until I have heard the evidence?'

Commentary

This story, the only one intended to be humorous which can be found by the editorial team despite exhaustive searching, highlights the appropriate question that should always be asked when any proposition is made: 'How do I know until I have heard the evidence?' However, hearing the evidence alone is insufficient. It is always important to make judgements about quality. A witness may be able to recount an impressive version of what happened but if s/he is not reliable then the evidence will be of little use.

CHAPTER 5

APPRAISING THE QUALITY OF RESEARCH

5.1 WHAT IS RESEARCH?

Research is a process of enquiry that produces knowledge. It is related to other activities, such as audit, but has several distinguishing features. In the UK, in the NHS R&D Programme, these features are defined as follows:

- to provide **new knowledge** necessary for the improvement of the performance of the NHS in enhancing the health of the nation;
- to generate results that are **generalisable**, i.e. that will be of value to those in the NHS who face similar problems but who are outwith the particular locality or context of the research project;
- to have been designed to follow a clear, well-defined study **protocol**;
- to have had the study protocol **peer reviewed**;
- to have obtained the approval, where necessary, of the relevant **ethics committee**;
- to have defined arrangements for **project management**;
- to report findings such that they are open to critical examination and accessible to all who could benefit from them – this will normally involve **publication**.

Research may fall into one of two categories:

1. that which increases the understanding of health, ill health and the process of healthcare;
2. that which enables an assessment of the interventions used in order to try to promote health, to prevent ill health or to improve the process of healthcare.

These two categories of research are linked. The former provides a base of knowledge from which ideas can be generated for preventing ill health or managing disease more effectively and efficiently – this is sometimes called hypothesis-generating research; the latter is used to evaluate the effects of putting such ideas into practice – this is sometimes called hypothesis-testing research. In this book, the focus is primarily on hypothesis-testing research because this is of greatest use to decision makers.

There are two methods for testing a hypothesis:

1. observational;
2. experimental.

Frequently, there are disputes between the proponents of experimental research ('trialists') and the proponents of observational or qualitative research; however, the focus on areas of disagreement has hidden the fact that there are many areas of agreement. One letter published in the *British Medical Journal*, written in response to an editorial,[1] usefully summarised the contribution of observational research,[2] which should be seen as complementary to experimental research trials and not presented as a false dichotomy (Box 5.1).

Box 5.1   Important roles for observational methods (Source: Black[2])

1. Some interventions, such as defibrillation for ventricular fibrillation, have an impact so large that observational data are sufficient to show it.
2. Infrequent adverse outcomes would be detected only by RCTs so large that they are rarely conducted. Observational methods such as postmarketing surveillance of medicines are the only alternative.
3. Observational data provide a realistic means of assessing the long-term outcome of interventions beyond the timescale of many trials. An example is long-term experience with different hip joint prostheses.
4. Whatever those who question the value of healthcare interventions might think, many clinicians often will not share their concern and will be opposed to an RCT; observational approaches can then be used to show clinical uncertainty and pave the way for such a trial.
5. Despite the claims of some enthusiasts for RCTs, some important aspects of healthcare cannot be subjected to a randomised trial for practical and ethical reasons. Examples include the effect of volume on outcome, the regionalisation of services, a control of infection policy in a hospital, and admission to an intensive care unit. To argue that these topics could theoretically be evaluated by an RCT is of little practical help in advancing knowledge.

1. Observational research

In observational research, the researcher observes a population or group of patients or manipulates data about those subjects. The researcher may use only those data that are already available or may collect further data, either from interviews with patients or healthcare professionals or from datasets such as cancer registries and death certificates. Qualitative research (Section 5.8), surveys (Section 5.6) and case-control studies (Section 5.4) are all forms of observational research. Observations may be made of variations already known to exist among different professionals or services – sometimes called a 'natural experiment' – or they may be made as part of an evaluation of some change in the health service introduced by a manager, politician or commercial company.

2. Experimental research

In experimental research, the same intervention is performed as a result of planning by the researcher. The most powerful type of experimental study is the RCT (Section 5.3).

It should be noted that:

- cohort studies (Section 5.5) can be either observational or experimental;
- although systematic reviews can be performed on any type of research, the term is most often used to describe reviews of RCTs.

It is possible to build an economic appraisal into all of the research methodologies described above (Section 6.6).

This chapter has been designed to help decision makers within any health service appraise the common types of research. The suitability of different research methodologies for evaluating different types of intervention is summarised in Matrix 5.1 and that for evaluating different outcomes in

Matrix 5.1

Intervention	Type of research				
	Qualitative research	Case control	Cohort	RCT	Systematic review
Diagnosis			√	√√	√√√
Treatment			√	√√	√√√
Screening				√√	√√√
Managerial innovation	√	√	√	√√	√√√

Matrix 5.2

Outcome	Type of research					
	Qualitative research	Surveys	Case control	Cohort	RCT	Systematic review
Effectiveness of an intervention					√√	√√√
Effectiveness of health service delivery	√	√	√	√	√√	√√√
Safety	√	√			√√	√√√
Acceptability	√	√			√√	√√√
Cost-effectiveness					√√	√√√
Appropriateness	√	√				√√√
Quality	√	√	√	√		√√√

Matrix 5.2. Often, for a complete evaluation, the results from more than one type of research method need to be used.

References

1. SHELDON, T.A. (1994) *Please bypass the PORT*. Br. Med. J. 309: 142–3.
2. BLACK, N. (1994) *Experimental and observational methods of evaluation*. Br. Med. J. 309: 540.

5.2 SYSTEMATIC REVIEWS

5.2.1 Dimensions and definitions

In primary research, the focus is on patients or populations; in secondary research, the focus is on reviewing primary research.

A review might include only one type of research, such as a review of surveys of RCTs, or a combination of different research methods, such as one review of the literature on the relationship between abuse (sexual and physical) and gastrointestinal illness, in which an association between these two problems was revealed, which included surveys, case-control and cohort studies.[1]

Although reviews, including editorials, may be readable and convenient to obtain, they are often misleading, principally because they are unscientific.[2] They are usually based on:

• an incomplete database – usually taken from MEDLINE searches (see p 62); *reviews should be based on a systematic search for evidence, both published and unpublished, and the search strategy used should be included within the review);*

- a subjective abstraction of data from primary sources; *reviews should be founded on a systematic appraisal (Section 5.2.1) of the primary sources; explicit criteria should be used to evaluate each study and described in the review;*
- poor analysis in which a variety of techniques is used; *reviews should be based on the systematic use of analytic methods, for example, correcting for heterogeneity when appropriate.*

In addition to these common flaws in the compilation and analysis of systematic reviews, there is also the problem of a reviewer's attitude. Reviews have long been viewed as 'second class' research; in the UK, the compilation of reviews was not recognised as a legitimate activity in the Research Assessment Exercise until 1995. A research worker who might devote hours to polishing an article about primary research to be read by other researchers would, when preparing a review, take a handful of articles from a filing cabinet and throw them into a weekend bag. This attitude has had detrimental consequences, not only for science but also for the public health.

A systematic review has the following characteristics:

- it is based on a clearly defined search of the literature, preferably by hand;
- explicit criteria are used to appraise the quality of the papers reviewed;
- the findings are analysed using validated methods.

In general, the findings of any research study have to be appraised in the context of all the other research evidence on a particular topic; this also applies to large single RCTs.

5.2.1.1 Meta-analysis

In a systematic review, the data from individual studies may be pooled and re-analysed. This technique is called meta-analysis; a systematic review in which this technique is employed is sometimes also called a 'meta-analysis'. There are two types of meta-analysis, depending on the source of the data analysed:

- MAL meta-analysis in which the data are abstracted from published papers in the literature, i.e. data on groups of patients;

- MAP meta-analysis in which the data have been obtained by asking the authors of published papers for the original single patient data and by asking drug companies for unpublished data.

MAP meta-analyses are more accurate than MAL meta-analyses.[3]

Economic evaluation can be a component of any of the types of research described above (see Section 6.6).

5.2.2 Searching

When searching for a systematic review, there is a simple sequence of steps to follow.

Step 1: Is there a review in the Cochrane Database of Systematic Reviews (see Appendix I)? If not, proceed to Step 2.

Step 2: Is there a review in the Database of Abstracts of Effectiveness Reviews (DARE) (see Appendix I)? If not, proceed to Step 3.

Step 3: Search MEDLINE, EMBASE (Appendix I) and other specialist databases (Appendix I).

To search for systematic reviews in MEDLINE, the strategy set out in Appendix II is that recommended by the Cochrane Collaboration.

5.2.3 Appraisal

A systematic review of all the evidence available is always more reliable than any single piece of evidence; the review of the relationship between abuse and gastrointestinal illness demonstrates this.[1] However, any systematic review must be carefully appraised. A checklist of questions for the appraisal of systematic reviews is given in Box 5.2.

Box 5.2 Checklist for appraising review articles (Source: R. Milne, CASP, see Appendix IIIB)

A. Are the results of the review valid?

Screening questions

1. Did the review address a clearly focused issue?

   HINT: An issue can be 'focused' in terms of:
   - the population studied;
   - the intervention given;
   - the outcomes considered.

---

2. Did the authors look for the appropriate sort of papers?
   HINT: The 'best' sorts of studies would:
   - address the review's question;
   - have an appropriate study design.

Is it worth continuing?

Detailed questions

3. Do you think the important, relevant studies were included?
   HINT: Look for:
   - which bibliographic databases were used;
   - follow up from reference lists;
   - personal contact with experts;
   - search for unpublished as well as published studies;
   - search for non-English language studies.

4. Did the review's authors do enough to assess the quality of the included studies?
   HINT: The authors need to consider the rigour of the studies they have identified. Lack of rigour may affect the studies' results.

5. If the results of the review have been combined, was it reasonable to do so?
   HINT: Consider whether:
   - the results were similar from study to study;
   - the results of all the included studies are clearly displayed;
   - the results of the different studies are similar;
   - the reasons for any variations in results are discussed.

B. What are the results?

6. What is the overall result of the review?
   HINT: Consider:
   - if you are clear about the review's 'bottom line' results;
   - what these are (numerically if appropriate);
   - how the results were expressed (NNT, odds ratio, etc.);

7. How precise are the results?
   HINT: Look for confidence limits.

C. Will the results help locally?

8. Can the results be applied to the local population?
   HINT: Consider whether:
   - the patients covered by the review could be sufficiently different from your population to cause concern;
   - your local setting is likely to differ much from that of the review.

9. Were all important outcomes considered?

10. Are the benefits worth the harms and costs?
    Even if this is not addressed by the review, what do you think?

If meta-analysis comprises part of any review, the process of appraisal must be more stringent. Meta-analysis is a powerful tool; performed correctly, it produces helpful evidence consistent with but having narrower confidence intervals than that from single trials (see Section 6.1.3). However, a recent incident has highlighted the need for care. A review including meta-analysis was conducted by excellent workers who reached the conclusion that magnesium treatment for myocardial infarction was 'effective, safe and simple'.[4] In contrast, in a large RCT, known as ISIS-4 (the fourth International Study of Infarct Survival), it was found that magnesium was ineffective.[5] This example demonstrates not only the superiority of large RCTs over systematic reviews of small trials but also the limitations of meta-analysis.[6]

The results of meta-analyses should be treated with caution for two reasons.

1. Meta-analyses are often based on data from trials found by electronic searches of MEDLINE, which:
   - covers only about one-quarter of the world's journals (see p 61);
   - finds only those trials that are electronically indexed, about half of the total (see p 61);
   - finds only those trials that are published, which are usually biased towards the positive.[7]
2. The data from the trials included in a meta-analysis are often heterogeneous, that is, there are important differences between them. Although there are statistical techniques that can be used to minimise the effects of heterogeneity, it still presents a problem.[8]

The questions that need to be added to the checklist in Box 5.2 for the appraisal of reviews including meta-analyses are shown in Box 5.3.

Box 5.3   Checklist for the appraisal of review articles that include meta-analysis

- Was the searching technique limited to an electronic search of MEDLINE?
- Are the results of the trials all or mostly pointing in the same direction?
  A meta-analysis should not be used to produce a positive result by averaging the results of 5 trials with negative and 10 trials with positive findings.
- Are the trials in the meta-analysis all small trials?
  If so, be very cautious.[9]

In contrast, Cochrane Collaboration reviews are based on:

- hand searches of the literature;
- searches of journals including, and other than, those on MEDLINE;
- unpublished data where it is possible to include it.

5.2.4 Uses and abuses

Although the systematic review is the best source of evidence for decision makers, systematic reviews do vary in quality. The decision maker must use his/her intelligence and the guidelines given in this chapter to appraise the review, before considering its relevance to the 'local' population and the decision that has to be made.

References

1. DRASSMAN, D.A., TALLEY, N.J., ALDEN, K.W. and BARRIERO, M.A. (1995) *Sexual and physical abuse and gastrointestinal illness*. Ann. Intern. Med. 123: 782–94.
2. MULROW, C.W. (1987) *The medical review article: state of the science*. Ann. Intern. Med. 106: 485–8.
3. STEWART, L.A. and CLARKE, M.J. (1996) *Practical methodology of meta-analyses (overviews) using updated individual patient data*. Statistics in Medicine 14: 2057–79.
4 TEO, K.K., YUSUF, S., COLLINS, R. et al. (1991) *Effects of intravenous magnesium in suspected acute myocardial infarction: overview of randomised trials*. Br. Med. J. 303: 1499–503.
5. ISIS-4 COLLABORATIVE GROUP (1995) *ISIS-4: a randomised factorial trial assessing early oral captopril, oral mononitrate, and intravenous magnesium sulphate in 58, 050 patients with suspected acute myocardial infarction*. Lancet 345: 669–85.
6. YUSUF, S. and FLATHER, M. (1995) *Magnesium in acute myocardial infarction. ISIS4 provides no grounds for its routine use [Editorial]*. Br. Med. J. 310: 751–2.
7. EASTERBROOK, P.J., BERLIN, J.A., GOPALAN, R. and MATTHEWS, D.R. (1991) *Publication bias in clinical research*. Lancet 337: 867–72.
8. THOMPSON, S.G. and POCOCK, S.J. (1991) *Can meta-analyses be trusted?* Lancet 338: 1127–30.
9. EGGER, M. and SMITH, G.D. (1995) *Misleading meta-analysis: lessons from an 'effective, safe, simple' intervention that wasn't [Editorial]*. Br. Med. J. 310: 752–4.

The interested reader should also consult the database of references of trials and review methodology which is part of The Cochrane Library.

5.3   RANDOMISED CONTROLLED TRIALS

> 'The RCT is a very beautiful technique, of wide applicability, but as with everything else there are snags.'
>
> Archie Cochrane,
> *Effectiveness and Efficiency*, 1989

5.3.1   Dimensions and definitions

An RCT is the best way of evaluating the effectiveness of an intervention, but before an RCT can be conducted there must be equipoise, that is, genuine doubt about whether one course of action is better than another.

The individuals who might benefit from the intervention being studied are randomly allocated to receive that intervention or not; the latter form the control group and receive a placebo or the 'standard' treatment. All entrants to the trial are followed up in treatment and control groups. Those individuals in the treatment group remain in that group irrespective of whether they actually receive the intervention; for example, in a trial of breast cancer screening those randomly allocated to receive screening remain in that group even if they do not attend for treatment – this is called randomisation on an 'intention-to-treat' basis.

In some types of RCT, such as drug trials, it is possible for both doctor and patient to be 'blind', i.e. unaware of whether the patient is a member of the treatment group or of the control group – such a trial is known as 'double blind'. The assessment of outcome should be done by an assessor who is unaware of the patient's status; this is known as 'blind' assessment. All patients must be included in the analysis. These steps are taken to minimise bias, a systematic error that favours either the treatment or the control group. The error is referred to as systematic because if it occurs once it will occur repeatedly due to a flaw in the design of the trial.

The other type of error arising in trials is that due to chance, which is random. Trials must be carefully designed to ensure that they have sufficient *power* to detect a difference between treatment and control groups, if one exists, or to demonstrate that there is no effect if the treatment is ineffective (Box 5.4).

> **Box 5.4** Power rules
>
> • The smaller the effect expected in the treatment being tested, the larger the trial necessary to have sufficient power to detect it.
> • The larger the trial, the greater its power.

5.3.1.1 Mega trials

To detect a small improvement in health outcome, for example 5%, a very large trial is needed. Although at first sight it might appear that a 5% improvement is clinically insignificant, for common diseases, such as myocardial infarction, a 5% improvement is of great importance. Large trials can be designed to demonstrate these small differences; sometimes called 'mega trials', they have made a significant contribution to the management of cardiovascular disease.[1] In a mega trial, there may be as many as 20 000 individuals in the treatment and in the control group.

However, mega trials do have limitations.

• To demonstrate a difference, many hospitals and numerous doctors in several countries must participate in a mega trial.
• For mega trials to be practicable, the criteria for entering patients into the trial must be simple such that a wide variety of different types of patient may be included; this is in contrast to the restrictive entry criteria that can be applied in a small trial.
• Doctors in the various countries involved may use treatments other than that being studied; this may lead to any effect of the experimental therapy being obscured.[2]

These weaknesses inherent in the design of mega trials necessitate a rigorous appraisal of any findings.

5.3.1.2 Adaptive design when the stakes are high

A different set of problems arises when the effect of treatment is great. For example, if a new drug administered to people who have end-stage cancer either confers a large benefit or alternatively leads to death in 50% of patients, it would be inappropriate to withhold it from or continue giving it to further patients in the trial once there is evidence the drug has good or bad effects. In such a situation, adaptive design is used to ensure that such effects can be identified early and the trial adapted or discontinued as appropriate.

5.3.1.3   Patient preference in trials

A methodological development of particular importance is
the incorporation of patient preference into trials in which
the patient's participation in the process of treatment, and
therefore their motivation, is essential for the intervention
to be effective. In drug trials, patient preference is not a
significant factor (all the patient has to do is swallow the
pills), but in other types of treatment, for example, a study
of subcutaneous continuous infusion pumps in the
management of diabetes, patient preference needs to be
built into the design of the trial.[3]

5.3.1.4   'N of 1' trials

The 'N of 1' trial is a single-patient controlled trial used in
the specific circumstances of the care of a patient whose
condition, depression for instance, fluctuates widely and is
affected by a multiplicity of factors such that the effect of
treatment is difficult to assess.[4] In such a situation, after
consultation with the doctor, the patient might agree to an
'N of 1' trial. During the trial, personnel in the pharmacy
will switch the patient's therapy between active and
placebo treatments (preferably twice); neither doctor nor
patient is aware of the switches, i.e. they are 'blind'. The
doctor and patient will meet at review consultations, but the
assessment of treatment outcome is carried out by a third
party, who is also 'blind', i.e. not aware of when the patient
was receiving the active drug or the placebo.

5.3.2   Searching

In addition to using the search term for the particular
treatment or test that is the focus of the decision, specify the
retrieval of RCTs.

The gap between a skilled MEDLINE searcher's haul and
that of an experienced clinical searcher was described in
Section 4.1 (see Table 4.3). The type of search strategy used
by a skilled searcher is given in Appendix II, but even this
is best used with a trained librarian to help.

The problems usually experienced when searching for
trials, because of the limited coverage of MEDLINE and
imprecise indexing, are diminishing as the work of the
Cochrane Collaboration begins to take effect. Hand searching
of journals, including those covered by MEDLINE and other
databases, has revealed many more trials such that about

100 000 are now easily available via The Cochrane Library (Appendix I). Previously, only about 20 000 RCTs were findable on MEDLINE, even by the best searcher.

5.3.3 Appraisal

During the 1970s, although the RCT was regarded as the 'gold standard' for demonstrating the effectiveness of a therapy, there was a growing awareness that this research method also had limitations.

- A survey of 71 negative RCTs showed that the majority of these trials were too small, that is, had insufficient power, to detect important clinical differences, a fact of which the authors seemed unaware.[5]
- A study of 206 RCTs showed that randomisation, one of the main design features of an RCT necessary to prevent bias, was poorly reported. Moreover, in those trials for which randomisation was not described, the effect of treatment was exaggerated by an amount greater than the true effect of the treatment (Table 5.1).[6]

Table 5.1 Methodological quality and estimates of treatment effects in controlled trials (trials with poor evidence of randomisation were compared with trials with adequate randomisation) (Source: Schulz et al[6])

Methodological issue	Exaggeration of odds ratio (%)
Inadequate method of treatment allocation	Larger by 41%
Unclear method of treatment allocation	Larger by 30%
Trials not double blind	Larger by 17%

- Other design and analytic mistakes were also reported, which almost invariably introduce a bias in favour of the drug rather than the placebo treatment. In one review, it was stated that: 'Doubtful or invalid statements were found in 76% of the conclusions or abstracts [of 196 double blind trials]'.[7] Bias consistently favoured the new drug in 81 trials and the control in only one trial.[7]

The message is clear: the results of RCTs, like any other research evidence, need careful appraisal using explicit criteria.

There are many factors that have been shown to bias a trial, and various checklists of quality criteria have been produced,[8] which are usually of most use to research workers. Chalmers has identified the three most important factors as follows:[9]

1. inadequate randomisation;
2. failure to blind the assessor of outcome;
3. failure to follow up all the patients in the trial and include all the data in the analysis.

These criteria are epidemiological and can be used to assess the quality of a trial; other criteria can also be used to assess the size of the effect found (Box 5.5).

A final note of caution: beware of subgroup analysis. It is tempting for the authors of any trial or meta-analysis to analyse data from subgroups of patients to look for treatment effects, particularly if the overall result of the trial is negative. This technique, known as subgroup analysis or data 'dredging', is risky and the checklist in Box 5.6 should be used when appraising subgroup analyses that identify treatment effects.

Box 5.5 Checklist for appraising randomised controlled trials (Source: R. Milne, CASP, see Appendix IIIB)

A. Are the results of the trial valid?

Screening questions

1. Did the trial address a clearly focused issue?
   An issue can be 'focused' in terms of:
   - the population studied;
   - the intervention given;
   - the outcomes considered.
2. Was the assignment of patients to treatments concealed?
3. Were all of the patients who entered the trial properly accounted for at its conclusion?
   - Was follow up complete?
   - Were patients analysed in the groups to which they were randomised?

Detailed questions

4. Were patients, health workers and study personnel 'blind' to treatment?
5. Were the groups similar at the start of the study?
   In terms of other factors that might affect the outcome such as age, sex, social class.
6. Aside from the experimental intervention, were the groups treated equally?

B. What are the results?

7. How large was the treatment effect?
   What outcomes were measured?
8. How precise was the estimate of the treatment effect?
   What are its confidence limits?

> **Box 5.6**   Guidelines for deciding whether apparent differences in subgroup response are real (Source: Oxman and Guyatt[10])
>
> 1. Is the magnitude of the difference clinically important?
> 2. Was the difference statistically significant?
> 3. Did the hypothesis precede rather than follow the analysis?
> 4. Was the subgroup analysis one of a small number of hypotheses tested?
> 5. Was the difference suggested by comparisons within rather than between studies?
> 6. Was the difference consistent across studies?
> 7. Is there indirect evidence that supports the hypothesized difference?

5.3.4   Interpretation and presentation

A research-based fact is like an uncut diamond, valuable but of little use. The decision maker has to be able to apply that fact. A checklist of questions that can be used to determine the applicability of research findings is shown in Box 5.7.

However, the application of any research evidence is difficult because the results from an RCT done on a sample of the whole population must be extrapolated to the population for which the decision maker is responsible; this involves judgements. It is important to recognise that there are two pervasive but subtle influences that bear upon a decision-maker's judgement and the way in which s/he might apply research findings to a 'local' population.

1. Cultural effects – interpretation
Cultural factors influence the interpretation of research evidence. In general, physicians in the USA have been quicker to adopt innovations in high technology than their counterparts in the UK. This difference is exemplified by the differing attitudes towards clotbusting agents.[11] It can be seen from Fig. 5.1 that tissue plasminogen activator (tPA) is no more effective than streptokinase, which is 10 times cheaper. Streptokinase also has fewer adverse effects, as shown in Fig. 5.2.

> **Box 5.7**   Checklist for assessing the applicability of research findings
>
> - How wide are the confidence intervals?
> - What were the exclusion and inclusion criteria?
> - How similar were the patients in the trial to the 'local' patient group?
> - Could the quality of service provided in the trial be reproduced 'locally'?

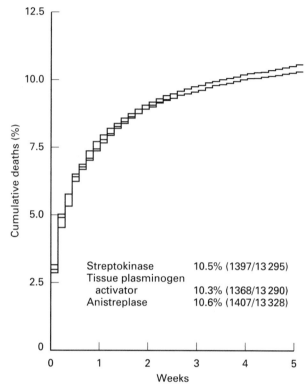

Fig. 5.1
Mortality of three agents compared in ISIS-3 (Source: O'Donnell[11], with permission, BMJ Publishing Group)

In the USA, tPA is the drug of choice; in the UK, it is streptokinase. American culture fosters the attitude that a novel intervention should be tried if there is no evidence against its use, whereas the attitude in the UK is that a new intervention should not be introduced until there is strong evidence in favour of its use: New World *vs* Old; Gung-ho *vs* Stick-in-the-Mud.

2. The framing effect – presentation (see Box 5.8)
If a picture is set off by a good frame, it will sell more easily – an evidence-based aphorism from the antiques trade. The same applies to research findings: decision makers are influenced not only by the data but also by the way in which those data are presented. This phenomenon, known as the framing effect, has been recognised by psychologists for years. It is used, consciously and unconsciously, by the pharmaceutical industry to present data in ways most likely to impress a clinician.

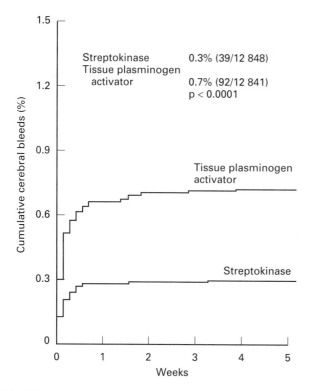

Fig. 5.2
Rates of cerebral bleeds with streptokinase and tissue plasminogen activator in ISIS-3 (Source: O'Donnell[11], with permission, BMJ Publishing Group)

Evidence of the existence of the framing effect is growing. The results of studies in Canada[12] and Italy[13] have shown the degree to which clinicians are influenced by relative risk reduction. This effect has also been shown to influence purchasers. Fahey et al[14] presented 182 health authority members with the results from a randomised trial on breast cancer screening and those from a systematic review on cardiac rehabilitation. The results were presented in four different ways as shown in Table 5.2.

Table 5.2 (Source: Fahey et al[14])

Information presentation	Mammography	Cardiac rehabilitation
Relative risk reduction	34%	20%
Absolute risk reduction	0.06%	3%
Percentage of event-free patients	99.82% vs 99.8%	84% vs 87%
Number needed to treat (NNT)	1592	31

Box 5.8   Aphorisms about data presentation in terms of relative risk

- For those who want to influence others, use relative risk reduction as the means of presenting data.
- For those who are likely to be influenced by data presentation, never, ever, accept information on the basis of relative risk reduction alone.

From the 140 questionnaires returned, it could be seen that the willingness to fund either programme was influenced significantly by the way in which the results were presented. Relative risk reduction stimulated a significantly higher inclination to purchase, followed by NNT. It is intriguing to note that only three respondents, 'all non-executive members claiming no training in epidemiology', recognised that the four sets of data summarised the same results.

References

1. YUSUF, S., COLLINS, R. and PETO, T.R. (1984) *Why do we need some large sample randomised trials?* Statistics in Medicine 3: 409–20.
2. WOODS, K.L. (1995) *Mega-trials and the management of myocardial infarction.* Lancet 346: 611–14.
3. BREWIN, C.R. and BRADLEY, C. (1989) *Patient preferences and randomised controlled trials.* Br. Med. J. 299: 313–15.
4. GUYATT, G., SACKETT, D., TAYLER, W., CHANG, J., ROBERTS, R. and PUGSLEY, S. (1986) *Determining optimal therapy – randomised trials in individual patients.* New Eng. J. Med. 314: 889–92.
5. FREIMAN, J.A., CHALMERS, T.C., SMITH, H. and KUEBLER, R.R. (1978) *The importance of Beta, the type II error, and sample size in the design and interpretation of the randomised controlled trial.* New Eng. J. Med. 299: 690–4.
6. SCHULZ, K.F., CHALMERS, I., HAYES, R.J. and ALTMAN, D.G. (1995) *Empirical evidence of bias: dimensions of methodological quality associated with estimates of treatment effects in controlled trials.* JAMA 273: 408–12.
7. GØTZSCHE, P.C. (1989) *Methodology and overt and hidden bias in reports of 196 double blind trials of non-steroidal anti-inflammatory drugs in rheumatoid arthritis.* Controlled Clinical Trials, 10: 31–56.
8. STANDARDS OF REPORTING TRIALS GROUP (1994) *A proposal for structured reporting of randomised controlled trials.* JAMA 272: 1926–31.
9. CHALMERS, I. (1995) *'Applying overviews and meta-analyses at the bedside': discussion.* J. Clin. Epidemiol. 48: 67–70.
10. OXMAN, A.D. and GUYATT, G.H. (1992) *A consumer's guide to subgroup analyses.* Ann. Intern. Med. 116: 78–84.
11. O'DONNELL, M. (1991) *The battle of the clotbusters.* Br. Med. J. 302: 1259–61.
12. NAYLOR, C. D., CHEN, E. and STRAUSS, B. (1992) *Measured enthusiasm: does the method of reporting trial results alter perceptions of therapeutic effectiveness?* Ann. Intern. Med. 117: 916–21.
13. BOBBIO, M., DEMICHELIS, B. and GIUSTETTO, G. (1994) *Completeness of reporting trial results: effect on physicians' willingness to prescribe.* Lancet 343: 1209–11.
14. FAHEY, T., GRIFFITHS, S. and PETERS, T. J. (1995) *Evidence-based purchasing: understanding results of clinical trials and systematic reviews.* Br. Med. J. 311: 1056–60

5.4 CASE-CONTROL STUDIES

For two decades, the case-control study was eclipsed by the RCT as the 'gold standard' in the evaluation of effectiveness, but in the 1990s its distinct and essential contribution is regaining recognition.

5.4.1 Dimensions and definitions

A case-control study is one in which the individuals selected for the control group have the same characteristics as the subjects of the study, except, that is, for the characteristic which is the subject of the hypothesis. In a case-control study of a cancer, for example, the subjects are those who have the cancer and the characteristics of these subjects, e.g. age, gender and smoking status, are matched with those of the controls, with the exception that those in the control group do not have cancer. In contrast, a study in which those who receive an intervention, for example, prostate cancer screening, simply by virtue of being eligible for a private service are compared with men of the same age who have not had the screening test because they were not eligible is not a case-control study: it is a badly designed and invalid trial.

A case-control study can be used to investigate the following problems.

- To study the causation of a disease. In a case-control study of people who had lung cancer it was found that smoking was the main cause of lung cancer: a large proportion of those who had lung cancer smoked whereas only a very small proportion of the control group, who did not smoke, developed lung cancer.[1]
- To identify the adverse effects of treatment. As the beneficial effects of treatment are usually more common than the adverse effects, a trial with sufficient power to detect the beneficial effects will probably not be powerful enough to detect adverse effects. Adverse effects can be detected either by following patients over many years in a cohort study (Section 5.5) or within a case-control study (Section 5.4). In a study of the adverse effects of treatment for high blood pressure,[2] 623 hypertensive patients who were members of a group health co-operative and who had had a first fatal or first non-fatal myocardial infarction were compared with 2032 hypertensive patients matched for age, sex and calendar year who

had not had a myocardial infarction. The following patients were excluded: those who had been members of the co-operative for less than 1 year; those who did not have a diagnosis of hypertension; those who had had a prior myocardial infarction; those whose infarction had been a complication of a procedure or surgery. Furthermore, patients entered into the study had to have been taking antihypertensive medicines for at least 30 days – preliminary analysis had shown that the recent starting of beta-blockers and calcium-channel blockers was strongly associated with a risk of myocardial infarction. Initial analysis included only those patients who were free of clinical cardiovascular disease. A strong association between acute myocardial infarction and dose of calcium-channel blocker, administered either alone or in combination with a diuretic, was found. The risk at the highest doses of calcium-channel blockers was three times that at the lowest doses. It is interesting that the authors of this case-control study then performed a systematic review of RCTs;[3] this underlines the need to evaluate a therapy using several different research methods.

5.4.2 Searching

Usually, the first step in any search strategy is to search for RCTs (Section 5.3.2). However, as the results of RCTs alone will not necessarily give all the outcomes of an intervention it is always useful to search for case-control studies.

5.4.3 Appraisal

Case-control studies have several advantageous features:

- they can be less expensive than trials (although some case-control studies are expensive because they involve a large number of subjects);
- they can sometimes be completed relatively quickly.

However, they are prone to bias: in a major review of case-control studies, 35 different sources of bias were identified.[4] For the user of research evidence or a decision maker, these 35 sources of bias can be distilled into two questions.

1. Was the selection of control subjects based on a set of criteria that matched the controls with the case subjects on every criterion except the presence of the disease or risk factor being studied?
2. Were measurements on the control subjects free from bias?

5.4.4 Uses and abuses

The main uses of case-control studies are:

- to identify the causes of disease;
- to identify rare effects of treatment, usually side-effects.

The main abuse of a case-control study is to evaluate the effectiveness of an intervention. The appropriate methodology to use in this situation is an RCT.

References

1. DOLL, R. and HILL, A.B. (1952) *The study of the aetiology of carcinoma of the lung.* Br. Med. J. ii: 1271–86.
2. PSATY, B.M., HECKBERT, S.R., KOEPSELL, T.D. et al. (1995) *The risk of myocardial infarction associated with antihypertensive drug therapies.* JAMA 274: 620–5.
3. FURBERG, C.D. PSATY, B.M. and MEYER, J.V. (1995) *Nifedipine. Dose-related increase in mortality in patients with coronary heart disease.* Circulation 92: 1326–31.
4. SACKETT, D.L. (1979) *Bias in analytic research.* J. Chron. Dis. 32: 51–63.

5.5 COHORT STUDIES

5.5.1 Dimensions and definitions

In a cohort study, a group of people is investigated over a particular period of time; any changes that occur during that period are recorded. A cohort study can be either retrospective, for example, reviewing all cases of three types of cancer in seven Californian hospitals between 1980 and 1982,[1] or prospective, that is, identifying a group of healthy people or patients and following them from one point in time to another.

In a cohort study, subject data may be those collected routinely or those collected specifically for the purpose of the study, or both.

A cohort study can be used to investigate the following problems.

- The outcome of treatment when, for ethical reasons, it is not possible to perform an RCT, for example, a study to determine the outcome of intensive care or prostatectomy.[2] The findings from this type of study enable quality standards, for example, the readmission rate,[3] to be based on evidence.
- Different approaches to service delivery and management when these cannot be tested by an RCT, either because the number of units is too small to confer adequate power upon the trial or because health service policy makers or managers will not allow their service to be included in such a trial. Cohort studies are also useful for the study of 'natural experiments', that is, when changes are made in the organisation or delivery of healthcare for political or managerial reasons or where different patterns of care exist in similar settings by reason of history and tradition. Cohort studies have been used to investigate:
  - staffing changes: for example, the effect of introducing on-site physician staffing to intensive care units in hospitals other than teaching centres (survival improved among patients who had an intermediate likelihood of death);[4]
  - the relationship between volume and quality (there is an association for some types of intervention, particularly those that are more complex);[5, 6]
  - the relationship between status and organisation of a hospital (e.g. teaching *vs* non-teaching, public *vs* private) and clinical outcome (although these relationships are complicated, important results can be obtained: for example, a 'positive correlation between higher mortality rates and hospitals located in States with strict prospective reimbursement programs' was found[7]);
  - the relationship between the organisation of a clinical service and clinical outcome (better co-ordination was shown to be associated with lower mortality in intensive care;[8] the admission of severely injured patients directly to an operating theatre was shown to reduce 'mortality, morbidity and suffering' in one cohort of patients who were followed for 9 years after a change in hospital organisation[9]);
  - the relationship between professional qualification and clinical outcome (although higher levels of qualification were associated with better outcome in one study,[5] this may reflect a failure to train the less highly qualified adequately).

Although it is possible to organise RCTs to assess the benefits of different types of service, such as a geriatric assessment service,[10] or of different methods of healthcare financing (for example, in one RCT the clinical outcomes of a health maintenance organisation and of a fee for service organisation were compared[11]), for many questions about the relationship between the funding and organisation of healthcare and patient outcomes, a well-conducted cohort study is the most appropriate form of research design.

In the funding or commissioning of research, the balance between promoting direct experimentation, through RCTs, and supporting observational studies, such as a survey of 'high cost patients in 17 acute-care hospitals',[12] has to be reviewed continually.

5.5.2 Searching

It is not necessary to search specifically for cohort studies. A search undertaken in the subject of interest will uncover them.

5.5.3 Appraisal

A checklist of questions that can be used in the appraisal of the findings of any cohort study is shown in Box 5.9.

Box 5.9 Checklist for appraising cohort studies

- Is clear information given about the way in which the cohort was recruited?
- Were any factors that could have included or excluded more severe cases considered?
- If mortality is a criterion, what steps were taken to ensure that all deaths were identified?
- If other criteria were used, have the instruments used for measurement been validated?
- Was the severity of disease taken into account in the analysis?
- Was the presence of other diseases (co-morbidity) taken into account in the analysis?

There are three study design features which are pivotal in the outcome of any appraisal.

1. The recruitment of individuals

The most important aspect of recruitment is completeness: all of the subjects in a defined time period should be recruited. Any sampling procedure applied to recruitment, such as the recruitment of patients who were admitted either on weekdays or between 0900 and 1700 hours, should create suspicion that the study results are biased. It can also be useful to ask: 'What happened to the patients who were not recruited?' It may be that the more severe cases were referred elsewhere or those undertaking referral may have referred only mild cases to the hospitals in the study.

2. Study criteria

The criteria used to assess the outcomes of care must be valid. For example, in-patient mortality is not a valid criterion of the quality of hospital care because of variations in duration of patient stay; it is better to use a criterion such as 30- or 60-day mortality. If criteria other than mortality are used, the techniques used to measure variables, such as pain or quality of life, should be validated.

3. Analysis of results

In the analysis of results, the severity of illness should always be taken into account and receive explicit mention in the paper. For example, in studies of intensive care, there is a validated system for assessing the severity of a patient's condition, known as APACHE (acute physiology and chronic health evaluation).[8] It is also important to control for the effects of co-morbidity, that is, the presence of other diseases that might have influenced outcome.[1] Robust techniques have been developed to do this and must have been applied to the clinical outcome if the results are to be accepted as valid.[13–15]

5.5.4   Uses and abuses

It is appropriate to use cohort studies to assess changes in health service management or organisation or to identify uncommon or adverse effects of treatment. The main abuse of a cohort study is to assess the effectiveness of a particular intervention when a more appropriate method would be an RCT.

References

1. GREENFIELD S., ARONOW H.U., ELASHOFF, R.M. and WATANABE, D. (1988) *Flaws in mortality data. The hazards of ignoring comorbid disease.* JAMA 260: 2253–5.
2. FOWLER, F.J., WENNBERG, J.E., TIMOTHY, R.P., BARRY, M.J., MULLEY, A.G. Jr. and HANLEY, D. (1988) *Symptom status and quality of life following prostatectomy.* JAMA 259: 3018–22.
3. HENDERSON, J., GOLDACRE, M.J., GRAVENEY, M.J. and SIMMONS, H.M. (1989) *Use of medical record linkage to study readmission rates.* Br. Med. J. 299: 709–13.
4. THEODORE, C.M., PHILLIPS, M.C., SHAW, L., COOK, E.F., NATANSON, C. and GOLDMAN, L. (1984) *On-site physician staffing in a community hospital intensive care unit.* JAMA 252: 2023–7.
5. KELLY, J.V., and HELLINGER, F.J. (1986) *Physician and hospital factors associated with mortality of surgical patients.* Medical Care 24: 785–800.
6. KELLY, J.V. and HELLINGER, F.J. (1987) *Heart disease and hospital deaths: an empirical study.* Health Services Res. J. 22: 369–95.
7. SHORTELL, S.M. and HUGHES, E.F.X. (1988) *The effects of regulation, competition and ownership on mortality rates among hospital inpatients.* New J. Med. 318: 1100–7.
8. KNAUS, W.A., DRAPER, E.A., DOUGLAS, M.S. and ZIMMERMAN, J.E. (1986) *An evaluation of outcome from intensive care in major medical centers.* Ann. Intern. Med. 104: 410–8.
9. FISCHER, R.P., JELENSE, S. and PERRY, J.F. Jr. (1978) *Direct transfer to operating room improves care of trauma patients.* JAMA 240: 1731–2.
10. STUCK, A.E., SIU, A.L., WIELAND, G.D., ADAMS, J. and RUBENSTEIN, L.Z. (1993) *Comprehensive geriatric assessment: a meta-analysis of controlled trials.* Lancet 342: 1032–6.
11. WARE, J.E., RODGERS, W.H., DAVIES, A.R. et al. (1986) *Comparison of health outcomes at a health maintenance organisation with those of fee-for-service care.* Lancet i: 1017–22.
12. SCHROEDER, S.A., SHOWSTACK, J.A. and ROBERTS, H.E. (1979) *Frequency and clinical description of high-cost patients in 17 acute-care hospitals.* New Eng. J. Med. 300: 1306–9.
13. KNAUS, W.A. and NASH, D.B. (1988) *Predicting and evaluating patient outcomes.* Ann. Intern. Med. 109: 521–2.
14. SEAGROATT, V. and GOLDACRE, M.J. (1994) *Measures of early postoperative mortality beyond hospital fatality rates.* Br. Med. J. 309: 361–5.
15. JENCKS, S.F. and DOBSON, A. (1987) *Refining case-mix adjustment. The research evidence. [Special article]* New Eng. J. Med. 317: 679–86.

5.6   SURVEYS

A survey is an investigation of what is happening at a point in, or within one period of, time. For example, in a survey of 61 US hospitals, in which the quality improvement approaches used in those hospitals were investigated in relation to an objective measure of clinical efficiency (length of stay), it was found that the most important determinant of quality was the management culture within a hospital rather than the specific quality improvement techniques utilised.[1]

A survey is a useful method of studying complicated situations; it can be combined with statistical analyses to increase its power. For example, in a study of the factors that promoted or hindered physician satisfaction with the hospital in which they worked, regression analysis was conducted on the survey results.[2]

However, the best way to increase the validity of a survey is to repeat it either after a period of time has elapsed or after some intervention has taken place: this type of study in which a population of people, patients or service providers is followed over a period of time is called a cohort study (see Section 5.5).

References

1. SHORTELL, S.M., O'BRIEN, J.L., CARMAN, J.M. et al. (1995) *Assessing the impact of continuous quality improvement/total quality management: concept versus implementation.* Health Services Res. J. 30; 377–401.
2. BURNS, L.R., ANDERSEN, R.M. and SHORTELL, S.M. (1990) *The effect of hospital control strategies on physician satisfaction and physician hospital conflict.* Health Services Res. J. 25: 527–60.

5.7   DECISION ANALYSIS

In evidence-based healthcare, decisions are based on a careful appraisal of the best evidence available, but how is that evidence actually incorporated into the decision-making process? One approach is for the evidence to be included in the discussion of issues together with information on the resources available and on the needs or values of the population under consideration. It is possible, however, to be more systematic, not only by describing the evidence that must be taken into account but also by estimating the impact of taking any of the various options – this approach is called decision analysis.

5.7.1   Dimensions and definitions

Decision analysis is a technique that enables a quantification to be made of the effects or impacts of the different options involved in any decision. Most decisions are not a simple choice between option A or option B; option A and option B may have different consequences. The analysis of a decision can be expressed as a 'decision tree'. To construct a decision tree the correct computer software is necessary (elegant software exists for designing decision trees[1]). It is also important to base any decision tree on robust information about the natural history of the condition under discussion and good evidence on the effects of different interventions.

Once a decision tree has been constructed, in which the consequences of various decisions are displayed together with the probability of each event occurring, values can be incorporated. It is possible to ask patients or members of the public to attach values to the good and bad outcomes of a decision, otherwise known as the utilities and disutilities (personal costs), respectively. In Fig. 5.3, a decision tree for screening for Down's syndrome for a population of 100 000 pregnancies is shown.[2] Values were given to the outcomes by women who participated in the study as follows: 0 represents a healthy live birth and 1 a Down's syndrome live birth; miscarriage as a result of amniocentesis and a termination because of Down's syndrome each have a weighting of 0.3.

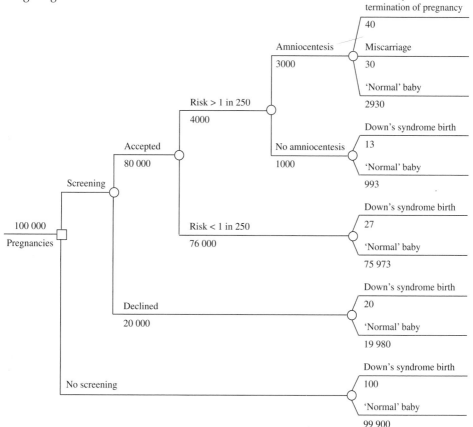

Fig. 5.3
Decision tree for Down's syndrome screening for a population of 100 000 pregnancies
(Source: Thornton and Lilford[2], with permission, BMJ Publishing Group)

To calculate the course of minimum expected disutility for any branch of the decision tree, the probabilities are multiplied by the disutilities. To take the example shown in Fig. 5.3: without screening, 100 Down's syndrome babies would be born. On the basis of various assumptions (shown in the figure), screening would detect 40 Down's syndrome babies (terminations) and 30 women would miscarry healthy babies as a result of amniocentesis. The expected disutility of a screening programme is:

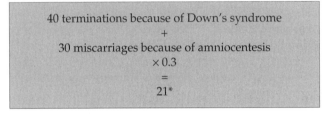

40 terminations because of Down's syndrome
+
30 miscarriages because of amniocentesis
× 0.3
=
21*

The expected disutility of not screening for Down's syndrome is:

40 Down's syndrome births × 1.0 = 40

Thus, screening results in a net gain of 19* 'utility units'.

The same technique can also be used to compare different screening policies. The decision tree in Fig. 5.4 shows the impacts of five different screening policies for detecting Down's syndrome before birth,[3] the decision analysis of which included financial cost but not disutilities. It also included sensitivity analysis which enables the effect of variations in one or more of the variables, such as the cost of ultrasound or the specificity of the serum test, to be examined.

5.7.2 Searching

Search for decision analysis articles using the term 'decision support techniques'.

5.7.3 Appraisal

A checklist of questions useful in the appraisal of the quality of a decision analysis is shown in Box 5.10.

Critical appraisal of a decision analysis can become intertwined with the core function of the decision analysis process itself. For example, criticisms of the decision analysis in which the impacts of various policies on Down's

---

* These figures have been corrected for a minor mathematical error in the published paper after consultation with Prof. Lilford.

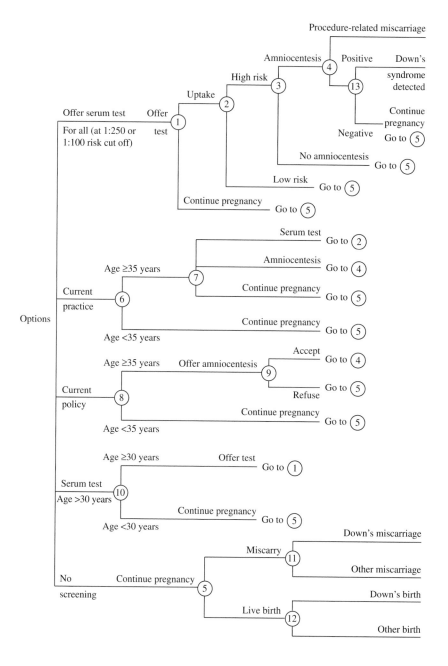

Fig. 5.4
Decision tree for five screening policies for detecting Down's syndrome before birth
(Source: Fletcher et al[3], with permission, BMJ Publishing Group)

syndrome screening were compared by Fletcher et al,[3] included the following:

- that the assumption of an uptake of 75% for amniocentesis was overoptimistic;[4]
- that age-specific values for sensitivity and specificity were not used;[5]
- that the costs were overestimated;[6]
- that the detection rates and the false-positive rates were too low.[7]

Although Fletcher et al dealt with these criticisms,[8] they pointed out that:

> 'One of the advantages of using decision analysis as a tool for considering the consequences of different screening policies is that the assumptions and numerical values on which the model's predictions are based are explicit. If there is debate about the assumptions or the numbers that should be used in the calculations it is easy to recalculate the model with the new numbers.'

A critical approach to decision analysis therefore does not necessarily reveal flaws in the technique but instead helps to clarify any assumptions that may have been implicit or 'fudged'.

Box 5.10 Checklist for the appraisal of a decision analysis

- What proportion of the branches in the decision tree represent good data based on good-quality research?
- If utilities or disutilities have been used, were they based on surveys of people with the health problem, surveys of a sample of the general population or estimates of the author's personal values?
- Has sensitivity analysis been performed to determine whether the estimate of effectiveness used in the decision analysis is higher or lower than the true level of effectiveness?
- Has sensitivity analysis been performed to determine whether the estimate of the incidence of side-effects is higher or lower than the true incidence of side-effects?
- Has sensitivity analysis been performed to test the analysis at estimates of financial cost higher or lower than the cost estimates used in the decision analysis?
- Has sensitivity analysis been used to test the effect of higher or lower utilities being assigned to different options?
- Have all the costs that should be taken into account been included?

5.7.4   Uses and abuses

Decision analysis should not be used to evaluate the effectiveness of an intervention; it should be used to give a decision maker an estimate of the impact an intervention may have on the population or group of patients for whom it is intended.

References

1. Smltree decision analysis software. J. Hollonberg, 16B Pine North, Roslyn, NY 11576, USA.
2. THORNTON, J.G. and LILFORD, R.J. (1995) *Decision analysis for medical managers.* Br. Med. J. 310: 791–4.
3. FLETCHER, J., HICKS, N.R., KAY, J.D.S. and BOYD, P.A. (1995) *Using decision analysis to compare policies for antenatal screening for Down's syndrome.* Br. Med. J. 311: 351–6.
4. MURRAY, D. and TENNISON, B. (1995) *'Decision analysis and screening for Down's syndrome.' Estimate of uptake of amniocentesis is overoptimistic (Letter).* Lancet 311: 1371.
5. SPENCER, K. (1995) *'Decision analysis and screening for Down's syndrome.' Not using age specific values invalidates study (Letter).* Lancet 311: 1371–2.
6. REYNOLDS, T.M. (1995) *'Decision analysis and screening for Down's syndrome.' Costs were overestimated (Letter).* Lancet 311: 1372.
7. WALD, N.J., KENNARD, A., WATT, H. et al. (1995) *'Decision analysis and screening for Down's syndrome.' Testing should be in all women (Letter).* Lancet 311: 1372.
8. FLETCHER, J., HICKS, N.R., KAY, J.D.S. and BOYD, P.A. (1995) *'Decision analysis and screening for Down's syndrome.' Authors' reply (Letter).* Lancet 311: 1372–3.

5.8   QUALITATIVE RESEARCH

5.8.1   Dimensions and definitions

Qualitative research can be used to gain an understanding of health and health services. The types of question best answered by qualitative research are shown in Box 5.11. The other types of research described in this chapter are

---

Box 5.11

- Why is it that people continue to smoke when the evidence about the harmful effects of smoking is all around them and known to a proportion of those who smoke?
- Why do people not take the medicine prescribed for them?
- Why do clinicians adopt innovations of unproven effectiveness while failing to adopt innovations of proven effectiveness?
- Why are nurses and doctors not able to work with one another with ease?
- What difference has the involvement of doctors in management made to the management of health services?

examples of quantitative research but qualitative and quantitative research both have a role to play in a science-based health service. Each research method is fiercely defended by its proponents but there is much common ground for agreement and increasingly health service professionals are beginning to understand that both qualitative and quantitative research are necessary.

Qualitative research has two main functions:

1. as part of a research programme that has a qualitative and a quantitative component. Sometimes quantitative research is preceded by qualitative work; for example, in the design of a study to identify the reasons why different services have different rates of intervention – in this case, it would be appropriate to conduct structured or semistructured interviews with lead consultants and managers to help design the quantitative research protocol. Similarly, in the preparation of patient questionnaires, it is often useful to discuss with focused groups of patients what they perceive to be the useful outcomes of treatment, otherwise outcomes chosen by clinicians and research workers might bear little relation to what is important to patients;
2. to complement quantitative research; for example, to capture information that complements data obtained from patient questionnaires, which can increase the validity of the information obtained by quantitative methods.

Qualitative research should not be regarded, however, as a method that merely complements and supplements quantitative research. It can often be used to generate hypotheses for the solution of a problem which can then be tested using either quantitative research, by building on the findings of the qualitative research, or a combination of qualitative and quantitative methods.

If the basic disciplines of quantitative research are epidemiology, biostatistics, psychology and economics, the basic disciplines of qualitative research are social anthropology and sociology. Although it is true that good managers use some of the principles of sociology and social anthropology in the performance of their job, qualitative research is different from the implicit and unconscious use of these disciplines because it is governed by:

- an explicit peer-reviewed protocol;
- ethics committee approval;
- a theoretical framework;
- a clear project management protocol;

- a means of identifying whether there are biases in the collection of information or drawing of conclusions.

5.8.2 Searching

It is not usual to search for qualitative research as a specific research type but qualitative research is often found when a literature search is conducted. As such, it is appropriate to focus on the appraisal of qualitative research.

5.8.3 Appraisal

The first step in appraisal is to determine whether the use of qualitative research in a study was appropriate.[1] The second step is to judge the quality of the qualitative research. As there are now good sources of information about qualitative research methods, it is possible to draw up criteria that can be used to judge quality. A checklist for the appraisal of qualitative research is shown in Box 5.12.

5.8.4 Uses and abuses

The main abuse of qualitative research methods is to appraise the effectiveness or safety of an intervention; in this situation, it is necessary to use quantitative methods. The main use of qualitative research is to gain an understanding of the working of any health service, which is particularly important to those who make decisions about groups of patients or populations.

Reference

1. MAYS, N. and POPE, C. (1996) *Qualitative Research in Health Care.* BMJ Publications, London.

Box 5.12   Checklist for the appraisal of qualitative research

- Was the research question clearly identified?
- Was the setting in which the research took place clearly described?
- If sampling was undertaken, were the sampling methods described?
- Did the research workers address the issues of subjectivity and data collection?
- Were methods to test the validity of the results of the research used?
- Were any steps taken to increase the reliability of the information collected, for example, by repeating the information collection with another research worker?
- Were the results of the research kept separate from the conclusions drawn by the research workers?
- If quantitative methods were appropriate as a supplement to the qualitative methods, were they used?

PROLOGUE 6

Dear Reader,

Empathise with the doctor. He had turned his head to locate the source of a greeting, and was shocked to find himself looking at what seemed to be a statue carved from Carrara marble: white sheets, cover, pillowslip, hair and face. 'How are you, doctor?' the occupant of the bed asked cheerily. The doctor struggled to recall the face, one of so many seen in a hectic year during the course of two busy surgical jobs. 'How are you?' said the doctor, dissembling well and still trying to recollect where he had seen the face before. 'I'm fine, doctor,' said the patient, 'but it doesn't seem like 5 months since I was last admitted. I've had such good care throughout.' Five months, last March, vascular surgery: the face came back but not the name. 'That's a long time,' said the doctor. 'Yes, but it's been wonderful whatever he's done, although I'm still trying to get used to this,' replied the patient waving his hand at the unnaturally narrow mound in the bed where two legs should have lain but where in fact there was only one.

Back in the ward office the doctor reviewed the case notes. The man had come in for a routine aortic graft. Although he had had symptoms of claudication they were not very severe. No-one had recommended the effective and safe therapy of exercise which should be standard practice before the knife is considered. The patient's first operation had been uneventful, but 7 days later he had thrown off a clot which had blocked the artery to his left leg; after two more operations the leg had been amputated. While recovering from the amputation he had developed a venous thrombosis in the remaining leg and suffered a severe pulmonary embolus. Whilst he was seriously ill from the pulmonary embolus, another clot had formed, this time in the artery leading to his intestine, and a portion of his intestine had had to be removed, giving him malabsorption.

He was now medically stable, waiting for a rehabilitation bed and a place in the unit where amputees are helped to adjust to and cope with the loss of a limb.

Commentary

Perhaps it is always unwise to speak of the outcome of care as if there is only one; there are very often many outcomes even though each clinician may see only one. The patient described in this prologue had thought that his initial operation was absolutely necessary and he was tremendously grateful for what he considered to be a life-saving act. The various clinicians who had seen him during his passage through the healthcare system had each had their own opinion as to the effectiveness, appropriateness and cost-effectiveness of the care he had been given and of the outcomes that had developed at each stage of this perilous journey.

CHAPTER 6

ASSESSING THE OUTCOMES FOUND

6.1 FIVE KEY QUESTIONS ABOUT OUTCOMES

Once it has been established that the research is of sufficiently good quality for the outcomes of the studies to be included within the framework of the decision, those outcomes must be assessed using five key questions.

- How many outcomes were studied?
- How large were the effects found?
- With what degree of confidence can the results of the research be applied to the whole population?
- Does the intervention do more good than harm?
- How relevant are the results to the 'local' population or service about which the decision is being made?

6.1.1 How many outcomes were studied?

The proposition that an intervention 'is effective' implies that there is only one outcome of care and only one objective in the design of that intervention. This is rarely the case. There are several outcomes of disease, and several beneficial outcomes of care are the corollary (see Table 6.1).

Table 6.1

Outcomes in the course of a disease	Beneficial outcomes of effective care
Death	Lower morbidity
Disability	Functional ability improved
Disease status deteriorates and risk of complication increases	Disease status, e.g. blood pressure, improves, risk of complications decreases
Dissatisfaction with process of care	Satisfaction with process of care
Distress about effects of disease	Feeling better

Although in Table 6.1 beneficial outcomes of care have been presented, the possibility that adverse effects may also occur must always be considered. It is the balance between good and harmful effects that should be weighed very carefully.

6.1.2 How large were the effects found?

The beneficial effect of a treatment for either an individual patient or a group of patients can range from 0% to 100%. For individual patients, benefit is measured by the magnitude of the effect, which ranges from no effect to complete cure. For a group of patients, magnitude of effect must also include the proportion of patients who will benefit, which is usually expressed as the odds ratio. The odds ratio is the ratio of the frequency of the key event, such as mortality, in the group receiving treatment to the frequency of the key event in the control group.

6.1.2.1 Which yardstick?

If a condition was previously untreatable, any new treatment must be compared with a placebo in trials. If, however, a treatment for the condition is already available, it is important to identify the difference between the effectiveness, safety, acceptability and cost of the two treatments. This may seem self-evident, but sometimes a difference in any of these criteria does not exist. Some research, particularly that funded by the pharmaceutical industry, is designed such that a new treatment is compared with a placebo irrespective of whether any therapies already exist; using this strategy, it is possible to give the impression that the new treatment is more effective than it actually is.

6.1.3 With what degree of confidence can the results of the research be applied to the whole population?

Research studies produce results, but these results are not necessarily the answer. Research is always conducted on a sample of the population of interest; even in a mega-trial of myocardial infarction in which 46 000 patients are enrolled, the 46 000 comprise only a sample of the millions of people who have a heart attack. Thus, a well-designed research study generates evidence of what happens only when the group of patients in that study are given a treatment;

it must not be assumed that the results of the study can be applied automatically to the whole population.

The degree to which the results of any study are generalisable can be expressed as a probability, both numerically and diagrammatically, using confidence intervals. The results of individual research studies are shown as single points in Fig. 6.1. However, each single figure result is only an estimate of the true effect as each study was done on a sample of the population. Although each sample may represent the whole population perfectly, the method of sampling always introduces errors. It is possible, however, to estimate the range of values within which the true result actually lies; this range is known as the confidence interval.

It is usual practice to calculate the 95% confidence intervals. These indicate that there is a 95% probability that the effect of treatment in the whole population lies within the range obtained and that effect is equally distributed on either side of the results obtained in the study population (see Box 6.1). An alternative way to express this is that there is a 1 in 20 chance that the effect in the whole population will lie outside this range. It is possible to calculate narrower confidence intervals, for example, 99%, but these often produce such a wide range of results that the preferred convention is to use 95% confidence intervals.

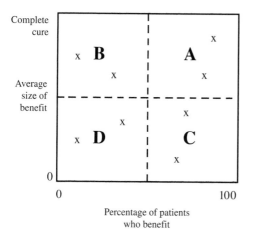

Fig. 6.1
Results of research studies. **x** represents the result for a single therapy; **A** represents good value, **D** poor value. If the effect is in either **B** or **C** the judgement is more difficult.

Box 6.1   Power rules

- The larger the sample of patients, the narrower will be the confidence intervals.
- The narrower the range of the confidence intervals, the greater the degree of confidence about the general applicability of the results.
- If both ends of the range of confidence intervals lie on the right-hand side of the line separating the beneficial from the adverse effects of treatment, there is a beneficial effect.

It can be seen from Fig. 6.2 that, for high-risk patients, even if the result of the review is, by chance, more optimistic than the true effect in the whole population, the intervention is effective because there is a clear benefit at the lowest end of the confidence intervals – point B. For individuals at low risk, even if the result of the review is, by chance, more pessimistic than the true effect, the intervention is ineffective because there is no benefit at the highest end of the confidence intervals – point C. For those at medium risk, it would be unwise to generalise from these results because the range in which the true effect lies includes both ends of the confidence interval, indicating that the intervention might be either beneficial or harmful.

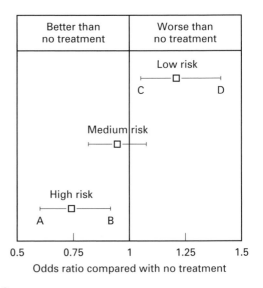

Fig. 6.2
Cholesterol-lowering treatments in individuals with different coronary heart disease risk

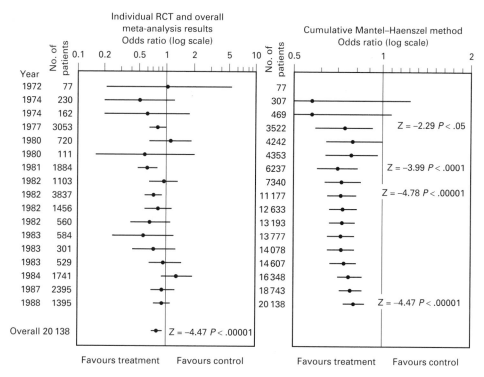

Fig. 6.3
Results of 17 RCTs of the effects of oral beta-blockers for secondary prevention of mortality in patients surviving a myocardial infarction presented as two types of meta-analyses. On the left is the traditional one, revealing many trials with non-significant results but a highly significant estimate of the pooled results on the bottom of the panel. On the right, the same data are presented as cumulative meta-analyses, illustrating that the updated pooled estimate became statistically significant in 1977 and has remained so up to the present. Note that the scale is changed on the right-hand graph to improve clarity of the confidence intervals (Source: Antman et al, JAMA, 8 July 1992, vol 268, p. 242. Copyright 1992, American Medical Association)

A cumulative meta-analysis, that is, an analysis that includes the data from all the trials as reported year on year, is shown in Fig. 6.3. It can be seen that the confidence intervals narrow as the numbers of patients included in the meta-analysis increase.

Although the increasing size of any trial narrows the confidence intervals, there is no need to design a mega-trial for every intervention tested because it is the size of the effect being forecast that determines the size of a trial; for instance:

- if a treatment is expected to cure someone with a disease that has hitherto been 100% fatal, only one patient is needed, as was the case with penicillin;

Box 6.2   Power rules part II

- The smaller the effect predicted, the larger the trial required to produce a result.
- The larger the trial, the greater the power.
- The greater the power, the narrower the confidence intervals.
- If the power calculations are correct and the size of the beneficial effect is as predicted, both ends of the confidence interval will lie on the same side of the line as the result.

- if a treatment might reduce mortality by 5%, thousands of subjects will have to be entered into the trial to demonstrate this effect (Section 5.3.1.1);
- if the effect of treatment might be greater than 5%, fewer patients will be necessary.

It is possible to estimate the number of patients required to ensure that a trial will be of sufficient size to produce a definite result. This is known as estimating the power of a trial (see Box 6.2 for the power rules).

6.1.4   Does the intervention do more good than harm?

When an intervention has beneficial effects, it is important not only to record their existence but also to indicate the probability of good or harm occurring. Few treatments benefit every patient and the balance of good and harm should always be estimated.

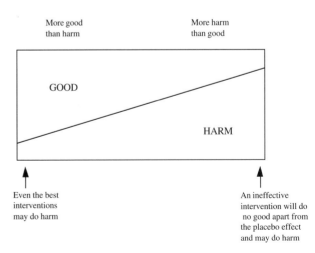

More good than harm

More harm than good

GOOD

HARM

Even the best interventions may do harm

An ineffective intervention will do no good apart from the placebo effect and may do harm

One of the many ways in which Scottish law is better than English is that there is a verdict in addition to 'guilty' and 'not guilty', that of 'not proven', a judgement of the strength of evidence. Similarly, in evidence-based healthcare, rather than classifying interventions as either 'effective' or 'ineffective', it is more accurate to classify them as:

- proven to do more good than harm – 'not guilty';
- proven to do more harm than good – 'guilty';
- of unproven effect – 'not proven'.

It must always be borne in mind that because an intervention has not been shown to be effective does not mean that it is ineffective, but neither can it be assumed to do more good than harm.

6.1.5 How relevant are the results to the 'local' population or service?

In protocols for research studies, especially trials, the criteria for inclusion and exclusion of patients are stipulated such that a homogeneous group of patients can be selected from which the intervention and control groups are randomised. However, this selection of a study population raises problems; for instance, how applicable are the results of a study of the treatment of heart failure in patients under the age of 75 years to patients over the age of 75 years? The use of less stringent inclusion criteria might decrease the proportion of patients excluded from the trial, thereby increasing the applicability of the findings, but it may reduce the validity of the trial. If certain results are considered to be applicable to the whole population, are they also relevant to any 'local' population which is the subject of a decision? Is a study of primary care in the Netherlands relevant to Northampton? Is the treatment given in a teaching hospital in Canada relevant to a district general hospital in Kent?

A checklist of questions that can be used to assess the relevance of research findings is shown in Box 6.3.

Box 6.3   Checklist for assessing the 'local' relevance of research findings

1. Does the population studied differ from the 'local' population in ways that are likely to be important with respect to:
   - genetic composition?
   - health status, e.g. is there a higher or lower prevalence of risk factors of disease in the 'local' population?
   - beliefs and attitudes, e.g. is the 'local' population likely to be more or less compliant with invitations to attend for screening?
2. Does the 'local' healthcare service have the potential to reproduce the service provided in the trial?
3. Could a similar level of resources as that available to the research workers be channelled into the 'local' service?
4. Are the skills to deliver a service of adequate quality available 'locally'? If not, is it possible to develop those skills at an affordable cost?

6.1.6   The clinician's conundrum

Dear Reader,

Empathise with Mr B. 'What do you think, doctor?' asked Mr B, who had been found to have narrowing of the arteries to his brain after investigation for a transient ischaemic attack. His GP had put him on aspirin and referred him to hospital. Mr B knew the aspirin was safe and effective and he had no trouble taking it. However, after numerous tests, the hospital doctor had advised him to have an operation on his carotid arteries – an endarterectomy – not unlike, he was cheerily told, rodding out pipes that had become furred up. So here he was, back in the surgery of his GP, whom he trusted, asking 'What do you think, doctor?'

Dear Reader,

Empathise with the GP. On being asked what she thought by Mr B, she was assailed by so many different thoughts. Why didn't consultants make the decisions? Isn't it just great to be a GP, trusted by both the patient and the consultant to whom the referral had been made! She thought of Mrs B, who had Alzheimer's disease: if Mr B has a stroke, she's had it. But there again he might not: not everyone with carotid artery stenosis does. What if he dies on the table? Some people do. What are the risks and benefits to Mr B? Where do I find the evidence? Why are these bloody difficult decisions always booked into a routine slot in morning surgery?

Commentary

Carotid endarterectomy is effective: it does more good than harm, but some people are harmed by the operation.[1] In fact, some of those who suffer harm would not have had a stroke even if they had not had an operation. It is essential for any clinician to know how to target treatment to individual patients who are at high risk of a poor outcome without treatment but who are also at a low risk of a poor outcome with treatment. In making this particular decision, the GP and Mr B were fortunate because an epidemiologist had actually completed and published the necessary research.[2]

For clinicians there is a further question: 'How relevant is this research to my patient?' The key issue a clinician has to consider is the 'baseline risk of the patient', that is, the degree of risk of a particular individual who shares the same characteristics as the patients in the trial.[3] Although this problem does not affect health service decision makers directly, they should be cognisant of the dilemma faced by the clinician and the patient: both individuals have to weigh up the probability of both good and bad outcomes occurring and the magnitude of the benefit and of harm.

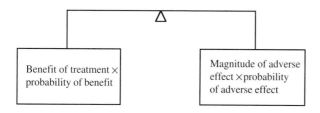

References

1. EUROPEAN CAROTID SURGERY TRIALISTS COLLABORATIVE GROUP (1991) *MRC European Carotid Surgery Trial: interim results for symptomatic patients with severe (70–99%) or with mild (0–29%) carotid stenosis.* Lancet 337: 1235–43.
2. ROTHWELL, P.M. (1995) *Can overall results of clinical trials be applied to all patients?* Lancet 345: 1616–19.
3. GUYATT, G.H., JAESCHKE, R.Z. and COOK, D.J. (1995) *Applying the findings of clinical trials to individual patients.* ACP Journal Club Mar–Apr; 122: A12–3.

6.2 EQUITY

6.2.1 Dimensions and definitions

One of the objectives of the NHS, explicit at the time of its institution and still implicit in many of its decisions, is equity. The definition of equity has occupied philosophers for years; there is no simple definition. However, equity is different from equality; for instance, no-one would argue that different patient groups should have equal shares of NHS resources. Equity implies social justice; fairness is one of the values on which NHS purchasing decisions are made.

Although social justice, or fairness, is felt keenly by everyone, can it be measured? Cost–utility analysis is a form of economic appraisal in which the quality-adjusted life year (QALY) is the outcome measure. It is possible theoretically to calculate the total number of QALYs provided for each patient group by a purchaser: if the QALY were the perfect measure of health benefit and if the purchaser had achieved perfect equity, the total number of QALYs for each patient group would be the same. This exercise has not been done as yet; it may prove impossible because of the amount of effort it would require and the imperfections inherent in the QALY.

6.2.1.1   Evidence-based cuts at the margin

There is one way in which evidence could be used to assess the equity of a purchaser's decisions: by analysis of the effects of marginal changes. If it were possible to identify the total amount of money spent on different disease categories (for example, eye disease, diseases of the ear, nose and throat, and diseases of the mouth), it would then be possible to determine the effects of either removing £500 000 from, or adding £500 000 to, each of those programme budgets. The effects of reducing spending on diseases of the ear, nose and throat by £500 000 could then be compared with the effect of increasing expenditure on eye disease by the same amount. This approach might prove useful in that it would narrow the debate about cuts to a relatively limited set of service changes; it would encourage decision makers to seek evidence useful in the quantification of the effects of such marginal changes on the population served.

6.3 EFFECTIVENESS

London has seen the birth of many revolutionary ideas, one of the greatest of which must be the National Health Service. This idea, first current in the 1930s,[1] was developed in many a draughty hall and lecture theatre. At one of these rallies, the young Archie Cochrane bore a banner carrying the slogan: 'All effective treatment must be free.'

The only reaction then, he reported,[2] was from someone who damned it for having Trotskyite tendencies. From this small beginning, the concept of effectiveness has become a major driving force for change in modern healthcare.

6.3.1 Dimensions and definitions

6.3.1.1 Effectiveness and quality

The effectiveness of a healthcare professional or service is the degree to which the desired outcomes are achieved. The quality of the service is the degree to which a healthcare professional or service conforms to preset standards of care (see Section 6.7).

The definition of effectiveness given above has not always been in use. Earlier definitions of effectiveness were broader and included efficiency;[3] today efficiency, or cost-effectiveness, is almost always used as a distinct criterion (Section 6.6), although it is not uncommon for the term 'efficient' to be used in the media when epidemiologists would use the term 'effective'.

6.3.1.2 Efficacy and effectiveness

The efficacy of an intervention is its impact in the best possible circumstances, whereas effectiveness is used to describe the impact of an intervention in everyday practice.

This is an important distinction because research is sometimes performed in an environment in which the level of resourcing and/or the number of skilled staff are greater than those available to the average service. For this reason, it is vital to consider not only the results of research but also the *relevance* of those results to the particular population or group of patients about which the decision is being made: an intervention may be efficacious at Massachusetts General Hospital, but will it be effective in the boondocks?

It is essential to evaluate effectiveness not only from a doctor's perspective, which is focused on death, disease status and, more recently, the functional ability of a patient, but also from the perspective of an individual patient.

6.3.1.3 The patient's perspective: feeling better and feeling happy

The delivery of effective and safe healthcare by professionals who are sensitive to the needs of a patient can engender the following emotional responses in the patient:

- the patient feels better about their health because effective care has brought about an improvement;
- the patient feels happy about the process of care because a sensitive professional has treated them as an individual.

The relationships of these two outcomes are presented in Matrix 6.1.

As can be seen, it is possible for a patient not to improve, or indeed to deteriorate, during the process of healthcare but still to be happy with the way in which care has been given (outcome B). It is also possible for a patient to feel better because the disease causing their problem has been dealt with effectively while feeling unhappy about the process of care (outcome C). The ideal outcome is D.

Patients whose health does not improve and who are unhappy about the process of care (outcome A) are difficult to assess; their view about the process of care may be influenced by the poor outcome for health status. Outcome A is the least satisfactory for both clinicians and patients.

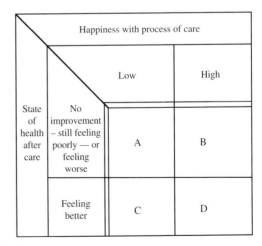

Matrix 6.1

Not only may health outcome influence the patient's perception of the quality of care, but the converse can also occur: the effectiveness of care, from a professional's perspective, may be increased if the patient's emotional needs are met by giving the patient support. This has been clearly demonstrated in an RCT of women in labour.[4] In comparison with the control group, the provision of emotional support by a professional or voluntary carer was found to:

- shorten the duration of labour;
- reduce the rate of Caesarean section;
- lessen the use of forceps;
- decrease the length of stay of infant hospitalisation.

The other important factor determining clinical outcome is the extent of participation the professional allows the patient in the process of care. In a controlled study, known as the 'friendly' dentists trial,[5] dental patients were assigned alternately to two 'treatment' groups: one group received care from dentists who were instructed to say things like 'Your opinion is more important than mine'; the other group comprised the control subjects and received care from dentists who behaved in the usual manner. It was found that outcome improved with patient participation.

The process of care is of greater importance when treating patients in whom there is no apparent structural disease but who have distressing symptoms, such as headache.[6] In this type of health problem, the nature of the process of care is the main factor determining the outcome.

6.3.2 Searching

To search for evidence of effectiveness, consult the following databases in the sequence shown.

1. The Cochrane Database of Systematic Reviews (Appendix I);
2. The Database of Abstracts of Reviews of Effectiveness (DARE) (Appendix I);
3. EMBASE and MEDLINE (Appendix I), for:
   - systematic reviews;
   - RCTs;
   - other types of study;
4. Specialist databases (Appendix I).

Use 'effectiveness' as a search term.

6.3.3 Appraisal

Evidence of effectiveness can be generated by several different types of research study. In the list below, the different research methods have been ranked in order of validity for obtaining evidence of effectiveness (the caveat is that all the research must be of high quality):

1. large RCTs (Section 5.3);
2. systematic reviews of RCTs (Section 5.2);
3. individual trials of inadequate size to detect adverse effects of treatment;
4. controlled trials without randomisation;
5. observational studies, such as cohort (Section 5.5) or case-control studies (Section 5.4), preferably from more than one research group;
6. the reports of expert committees, the writing of which has been based upon the sources of evidence cited and not simply the opinion of eminent committee members.

A checklist of questions for the appraisal of research evidence on effectiveness is shown in Box 6.4.

Once evidence has been found and its quality appraised, it is necessary to address the implications of the research findings (see Box 6.5 and Table 6.2).

Box 6.4   Checklist for appraising research evidence of effectiveness

1. Does the research provide evidence about adverse effects (Section 6.4) and the patients' perspectives of outcome (Section 6.5)?
2. What is the magnitude of the beneficial effect?
3. With what degree of confidence can the findings in a research setting be reproduced in ordinary clinical settings?

Box 6.5   The possible implications of evidence of effectiveness for the provision of healthcare in a 'local' service

- If the trial results are negative, that is, no effect is shown, and this treatment is being delivered within the 'local' service, search for other evidence because the treatment may not be effective.
- If the trial results are positive and this treatment is being delivered within the 'local' service, ascertain how large the effect is at what risk and at what cost. (The NNT is of use in this assessment.)
- If the trial results are positive and this treatment is not being delivered within the 'local' service, consider implementing the research findings but beware of the five positive biases (Table 6.2).

Table 6.2 Five positive biases

Bias	Cause
Submission bias	Research workers are more strongly motivated to complete, and submit for publication, positive results
Publication bias	Editors are more likely to publish positive studies[7]
Methodological bias	Methodological errors such as flawed randomisation produce positive biases[8]
Abstracting bias	Abstracts emphasise positive results[9]
Framing bias	Relative risk data produce a positive bias[10]

6.3.3.1 Experimental studies of effectiveness

1. The odds ratio: the relative benefit
The magnitude of the beneficial effect is often expressed in relative terms as the odds ratio.

- In a controlled trial, if the odds ratio is equal to 1, treatment has no effect.
- If the odds ratio is less than 1, the treatment has a beneficial effect when compared with the intervention applied to the control group.
- If the odds ratio is greater than 1, the treatment is less effective than the intervention applied to the control group.

For a lucid explanation of the odds ratio, follow the example given in the Cochrane Collaboration Handbook (for URL, see p 223).

The presentation of trial data in terms of relative risk introduces a bias: readers interpret the results as being more positive than they actually are – the framing effect (Section 5.3.4). It is therefore important to consider the absolute reduction in risk that a treatment will produce.

2. NNT: the absolute benefit
The number needed to treat (NNT) is a comprehensible measure of the absolute effects of treatment;[11] the NNT for various interventions-to-outcomes are set out in Table 6.3. The clarity gained by presenting data in this way is striking: only 15 people with severe high blood pressure have to be given treatment to prevent one stroke, but among people with mild hypertension 700 have to be treated to prevent one stroke.

Table 6.3   NNTs for some cardiac interventions (Source: extracts from *Bandolier* 1995; 17: 7)

Intervention	Outcome	NNT
CABG in left main stenosis	Prevent 1 death at 2 years	6
Carotid endarterectomy in high-grade symptomatic stenosis	Prevent 1 stroke or death in 2 years	9
NNTs for hypertension treatment		
Simple antihypertensives for severe hypertension	Prevent 1 stroke, MI or death in 1 year	15
Simple antihypertensives for mild hypertension	Prevent 1 stroke, MI or death in 1 year	700
Treating hypertension in the over-60s	Prevent 1 coronary event	18
NNTs for angina treatment		
Aspirin in severe unstable angina	Prevent MI or death in 1 year	25
Aspirin in healthy US physician	Prevent MI or death in 1 year	500

6.3.3.2   Observational studies of effectiveness

It had been hoped that routinely collected data on computer systems in a health service would enable the effectiveness of new technology to be evaluated within observational studies. Unfortunately experience has not lived up to early expectations. The principal reason for this is the absence of a 'control' group in this methodology. Consequently, it is impossible to know if the effects of treatment are generalisable or if they are due to factors such as the preferential selection of patients for one particular intervention as opposed to another. Large databases of outcomes cannot be used to provide definitive answers about effectiveness: as one authority states, 'while databases can suggest problems and offer answers, they cannot prove them; database analysis must be followed by trials.'[12]

The potential of and pitfalls associated with observational studies are exemplified by the investigations of the safety of prostatic surgery. Transurethral resection of the prostate gland (TURP) for benign prostatic hypertrophy became fashionable in the 1970s; by the mid 1980s, it was the operation in common use. In 1989, the results of an observational study indicated that TURP was associated with a higher long-term mortality rate than the traditional operation of open prostatectomy (OP) – an increase of 45%.[13] Other evidence against the use of TURP was also published.[14, 15] However, not all the possible reasons for this difference in mortality had been taken into account. In particular, during the analysis of the results, allowance was not made for the differences in selection criteria for men undergoing OP and for those undergoing TURP which pertain because of the increased short-term morbidity and mortality associated with OP. Once this had been taken into account,[16] the conclusion was very different from the increase in mortality from TURP previously reported; the author of this excellent study concludes that:

> 'The apparent excess in long-term mortality after TURP is unlikely to be caused by the operation itself. It is more likely to reflect relatively low long-term mortality in OP patients as a consequence of the OP patients having been relatively fitter than those having TURP'.[16]

Thus, it is not yet possible to convict TURP of causing excess mortality; any previous convictions were made on the basis of flawed evidence. Seagroatt also concluded that any differences in long-term mortality can be 'answered only in a randomised clinical trial', but emphasises that such a trial may be impossible to organise.[16]

6.3.4 Applicability and relevance

Confidence intervals provide the best guide to the applicability of research results. The narrower the confidence intervals, the more confident a decision maker can be that the research evidence represents the effect that it is possible to obtain in the whole population.

A checklist of questions for the assessment of the applicability and relevance of research evidence on effectiveness is shown in Box 6.6.

Box 6.6 Checklist for assessing the applicability of research evidence of effectiveness to the 'local' population and service

- Is the study population similar to the 'local' population:
  - genetically?
  - socially?
  - medically?

- Is the service or treatment under investigation similar to that available 'locally' in terms of:
  - skills?
  - resources?

References

1. WEBSTER, C. (1988) *The Health Services Since the War: Volume 1.* HMSO, London.
2. COCHRANE, A. (1972) *Effectiveness and Efficiency.* Nuffield Provincial Hospitals Trust, London.
3. DOLL, R. (1974) *Surveillance and Monitoring.* Int J. Epidemiol. 3: 305–14.
4. KENNELL, J., KLAUS, M., MCGRATH, S., ROBERTSON, S. and HUNTLY, C. (1991) *Continuous emotional support during labor in a US hospital.* JAMA 265: 2197–201.
5. LEFER, L., PLEASURE, M.A. and RESENTHAL, L. (1962) *A psychiatric approach to the denture patient.* J. Psychosom. Res. 6: 199–207.
6. FITZPATRICK, R. and HOPKINS, A. (1981) *Referrals to neurologists for headaches not due to structural disease.* J. Neurol. Neurosurg. Psychiat. 44: 1061–7.
7. EASTERBROOK, P.J., BERLIN, J.A., GOPALAN, R. and MATTHEWS, D.R. (1991) *Publication bias in clinical research.* Lancet 337: 867–72.
8. SCHULZ, K.F., CHALMERS, I., GRIMES, D.A. and ALTMAN, D. (1994) *Assessing the quality of randomization from reports of controlled trials published in obstetrics and gynecology journals.* JAMA 272: 125–8.
9. GØTZSCHE, P.C. (1989) *Methodology and overt and hidden bias in reports of 196 double-blind trials of nonsteroidal anti-inflammatory drugs in rheumatoid arthritis.* Controlled Clinical Trials 10: 31–56.
10. FAHEY, T., GRIFFITHS, S. and PETERS, T.J. (1995) *Evidence-based purchasing: understanding results of clinical trials and systematic reviews.* Br. Med. J. 311: 1056–60.
11. COOK, R.J. and SACKETT, D.L. (1995) *The number needed to treat: a clinically useful measure of treatment effect* Br. Med. J. 310: 452–4.
12. TEMPLE, R. (1990) *Problems in the use of large data sets to assess effectiveness.* Int. J. Technol. Assess. Health Care 6: 211–19.
13. ROOS, N.P., WENNBERG. J.E., MALENKA, D.J. et al. (1989) *Mortality and reoperation after open and transurethral resection of the prostate for benign prostatic hyperplasia.* New Eng. J. Med. 320: 1120–4.
14. ANDERSEN, T.F., BRONNUM-HANSEN, H., SEJR, T. and ROEPSTORFF, C. (1990) *Elevated mortality following transurethral resection of the prostate for benign hypertrophy! But why?* Med. Care 28: 870–81.
15. SIDNEY, S., QUESENBERRY, C.P., SADLER, M.C. et al. (1992) *Reoperation and mortality after surgical treatment of benign prostatic hypertrophy in a large prepaid medical care program.* Med. Care 30: 117–25.
16. SEAGROATT, V. (1995) *Mortality after prostatectomy: selection and surgical approach.* Lancet 346: 1521–4.

6.4 SAFETY

Arthur Dent:	'If I asked you where the hell we were, would I regret it?'
Ford Prefect:	'We're safe.'
Arthur Dent:	'Oh good.'
Ford Prefect:	'We're in a small galley cabin in one of the space ships of the Vogon Constructor Fleet.'
Arthur Dent:	'Ah, this is obviously some strange usage of the word safe that I wasn't previously aware of.'

Douglas Adams,
The Hitch Hiker's Guide to the Galaxy, 1979

6.4.1 Dimensions and definitions

Safety and risk are inversely related to one another:

Safety $= 1 -$ risk of adverse effects

The risk associated with an intervention is the 'probability' that an adverse effect will occur.

The use of the word 'probability' is interesting: most people use the 1576 definition, given in the *Shorter Oxford English Dictionary* as 'something which, judged by present evidence, is likely to happen', rather than the 1718 mathematical definition which is 'the amount of antecedent likelihood of a particular event as measured by the relative frequency of occurrence of events of the same kind in the whole course of experience'. Words used to describe frequency, such as likely, often, sometimes, possible and frequently, can be interpreted by different individuals differently. This difference in interpretation is also evident in expressions of 'subjective possibility' (*SOED*); for example, 'Side-effects may occur'. There are, however, generally held distinctions; for instance, that 'probable' implies a higher frequency than 'possible'. As the variation in the weighting given to different words is so great, numbers have to be used, but which numbers?

Risk can be expressed in two ways, as:

1. relative risk;
2. absolute risk.

Relative risk can be expressed in comprehensible terms: for example, 'Men randomised to the thiazide (for high blood pressure) were 20 times as likely as men on the placebo to be withdrawn from the trial because of impotence'.[1] Relative risk can also be expressed as a single number: to continue with the example, the relative risk of impotence in men who remain on the thiazide treatment for high blood pressure is 2.3, with 23% of men on thiazides being impotent after two years' treatment in comparison with only 10% of those receiving placebo.[1]

Absolute risk is used to express probability either as a simple percentage, for example, 'About 60% of patients will experience adverse effects', or the number needed to treat (the NNT – see Section 6.3.3.1). Some patients may find the NNT more comprehensible than a percentage. The NNT or, in this context, the NNH (the number needed to harm), i.e. the number of patients treated with thiazide diuretics that would result in one person being harmed over and above the risk in the general population, is 8. This figure, the NNI (the number needed to cause an extra case of impotence), is calculated by converting the relative risk to an absolute figure using the following formula:

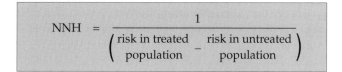

$$NNH = \frac{1}{\left(\begin{array}{c}\text{risk in treated} \\ \text{population}\end{array} - \begin{array}{c}\text{risk in untreated} \\ \text{population}\end{array}\right)}$$

As for all other outcome estimates, confidence intervals should be given.

6.4.2   Searching

Step 1. Specify the intervention in question: the drug, test or operation.

Step 2. Specify adverse effects or risk of adverse effects.

It is not normally useful to stipulate a publication type. Although the best evidence is provided by a systematic review of RCTs, other methods of research can also be helpful, so it is important not to limit the boundaries of the search in this way.

6.4.3 Appraisal

The first two steps in the critical pathway of appraisal are:

1. What is the best research method to give information about the risks of treatment?
2. How good is the quality of the research?

The three research methods that can generate evidence about safety and the risk of adverse effects of treatment are (in order of validity):

1. RCTs (Section 5.3);
2. surveys (Section 5.6) and cohort studies (Section 5.5);
3. case-control studies (Section 5.4).

Systematic reviews of any of these methods of research (Section 5.2) are better than single studies provided the quality of the primary research is good.

Randomised controlled trials that generate useful evidence about the harmful effects of treatment are relatively rare, principally because the adverse effects of treatment usually occur less frequently than the beneficial effects. A trial designed with sufficient power to demonstrate the beneficial effects of treatment (Section 6.1) will probably not have sufficient power to detect any adverse effects and it is often necessary to perform a cohort study.

A cohort study is a research design in which several groups of patients are followed over time: one group receives the treatment under investigation while one or more other groups act as controls. For example, thousands of British women who were and were not taking oral contraceptives have been followed for years. However, those women not taking oral contraceptives cannot be compared directly with those who are; although deep vein thrombosis may have been detected more often in pill users, the possibility exists that non-users may not have been prescribed the pill because they were considered to be at high risk of thrombosis anyway.

Prospective cohort studies are less prone to bias and can be used when it is not possible to conduct an RCT. For example, most anaesthetists might refuse to participate in an RCT to test the hypothesis that epidural anaesthesia causes backache. However, it did prove possible to follow 329 women for six weeks after delivery, 164 of whom had had epidural anaesthesia and 165 of whom had not. The results of this prospective study of these two cohorts did not show that backache was an adverse effect of epidural anaesthesia.[2]

Although the design of case-control studies may introduce a greater degree of bias than that of cohort studies, it may be the most appropriate study design to identify the adverse effects of drugs.

A major source of bias is introduced if data collected previously are reviewed. In an elegant experiment, 112 anaesthetists were asked to review 21 cases for which there had been adverse outcomes. The original classification of outcome was given as either permanent or temporary. The anaesthetists were also asked to review a further 21 cases that had been made up by the researchers to match the original 21 cases in every way except that the outcomes were interchanged: if the original case had a temporary impairment, the matched fictional case was given a permanent impairment, and vice versa. The results were startling: the proportion of ratings for appropriate care were *decreased* by 31% when the outcome was changed from temporary to permanent, and increased by 28% when the outcome was changed from permanent to temporary. From this study, it can be seen that knowing the outcome can alter the reviewer's perception of the safety of the care given.[3]

Although the quality of each type of research study must be appraised using the criteria set out in the relevant sections of the book, there are some general questions that should be used in the appraisal of any study designed to investigate adverse effects (see Box 6.7).

Box 6.7 Checklist for appraising the quality of a study designed to investigate adverse effects

1. Was the assessment of outcomes free from bias?
2. Was there an adverse effect greater than would be expected by chance, taking into account the confidence intervals?
3. How important is the adverse effect clinically?
4. If more than one study is available, are the results consistent between or among studies?

6.4.4   Applicability and relevance

Evidence revealing risks associated with drug treatment can usually be applied to the whole population: the results are relevant to all patients of the same type as those described in the original trial. In contrast, the risks associated with particular surgical operations or interventions, in which the skill of the professional is an important determining factor, may vary according to the professional involved; therefore, the risk may be smaller or greater than that reported in the literature.

A checklist of questions for the assessment of the applicability and relevance of research findings on safety is shown in Box 6.8.

Box 6.8   Checklist for assessing the applicability and relevance of research evidence of safety

1. Were the professionals participating in the study
   more highly specialised or
   more experienced in this intervention than those
   who will be treating the 'local' population?
2. Would the quality of training be important in
   determining the frequency of adverse effects?
3. Were the patients in the research study different
   from those in the 'local' population, either by being
   fitter or by having more advanced disease?

References

1. MEDICAL RESEARCH COUNCIL WORKING PARTY (1981)
   Adverse reactions to bendrofluazide and propanolol for the treatment of mild hypertension. Lancet ii: 539–43.
2. MACARTHUR, A., MACARTHUR, C. and WEEKS, S. (1995)
   Epidural anaesthesia and low back pain after delivery: a prospective cohort study. Br. Med. J. 311: 1336–9.
3. CAPLAN, R.A., POSNER, K.L. and CHENEY, F.W. (1991)
   Effect of outcome on physician judgements of appropriateness of care. JAMA 265: 1957–60.

Dear Reader,

Empathise with Mr R. He spat accurately into the bucket that served as both spittoon and urinal. Disabled by a stroke and a gas lung sustained in an afternoon during the First World War when the gas came 'rolling towards us', he was unable to climb the stairs to get to the bathroom of his damp council house. The room in which he lived was heated by only a small electric fire; mould had formed an opulent brocade on the walls. Although the young doctor and social worker were apologising for their inability to improve his health and environment, his views were clear. 'I'm grateful for all you're doing, but don't worry about me; I'm all right. Sixty years ago today I was up to my waist in mud and water.'

Commentary

Satisfied with his lot, satisfied with his services, this Old Contemptible would never have dreamed of complaining, but times have changed and patient satisfaction can no longer be taken for granted.

6.5.1   Dimensions and definitions

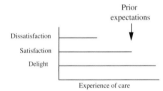

The level of a patient's satisfaction is directly related to the degree to which their expectations have been met.

However, satisfaction is an imperfect measure with which to assess the quality of a service: it is possible for patients to be delighted with healthcare in which the quality of clinical practice is poor if their expectations were low.

Moreover, the assessment of satisfaction, although necessary, is not sufficient: satisfaction is determined not only by the quality of the service but also by patient expectations. Therefore, it is necessary to assess the patient's experience of care and make a judgement about the quality of that experience irrespective of whether the patient is satisfied. As an example, a patient may be satisfied with the amount of information provided and the way in which it was provided, even if that information is wrong and misleading; it is essential, therefore, to complement the question 'Were you satisfied with the information you were given?' with the question 'What information were you given?' Increasing use is being made of systems designed to assess patient experience.

This novel approach, developed in the USA, to gather patients' experiences involves asking patients to report on how much pain they had or whether they had been informed about problems that might occur after discharge, for example.

This approach was used to improve medical care in 10 hospitals in the USA.[1] In the UK, a national survey of 36 NHS hospitals was undertaken which involved interviewing 5150 randomly chosen NHS patients.[2] Patients were asked direct questions about their experiences during their stay in hospital and not simply subject to a general enquiry about their level of satisfaction. The conclusion was that asking patients about what had happened rather than how satisfied they were with treatment gave a better understanding of what might be wrong with a service and provided a stronger base upon which to improve.

A patient's experience is determined by three inter-related aspects of care:

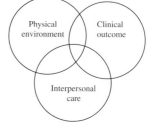

1. the clinical outcome;
2. the physical environment in which care is received;
3. the interpersonal relationships of care, namely, how patients are treated by carers.

6.5.1.1 Clinical outcome: expectations and experience

The relationship between the patient's and the clinician's perceptions of outcome was discussed on pp 114–5. Although a patient's expectations may be determined by many factors, such as what they have read or what friends have told them, the single most important factor is what they remember the clinician said about clinical outcomes, such as:

- the magnitude of health improvement that could be expected, e.g. complete cure or alleviation of symptoms;
- the probability that there would be a benefit;
- the side-effects that most commonly occur;
- the probability that any of those side-effects would be suffered personally.

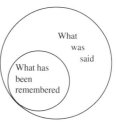

The optimal information exchange in a consultation is when the patient remembers all that the clinician said; however, this does not always occur. Thus, the most important factor is the quality of the clinician's communication.

	Beneficial effect as good as predicted and expected	Beneficial effect absent or not as good as predicted or expected
No side-effects	Delighted	Disappointed
Side-effects as expected or predicted	Modified delight	Very disappointed
Side-effects greater than expected or predicted	Response dependent upon personality and other factors, e.g. satisfaction with interpersonal care	Desolate

Matrix 6.2

The various reactions a patient might have are shown in Matrix 6.2.

Patients' reactions may also vary depending upon:

- factors over which the health service has no influence, e.g.
  - the patient's personality;
  - the advice of ambulance-chasing lawyers;
- factors over which the health service has influence, e.g.
  - the physical environment;
  - the quality of interpersonal care.

6.5.1.2 The physical environment: expectations and experience

Certain aspects of the physical environment in which care is delivered are of particular importance to patients:

- food;
- parking;
- cleanliness;
- the comfort of the bed;
- the 'external' environment (is it possible to see trees from the bed?);
- ease of access by public transport.

If the clinical outcome is satisfactory and the interpersonal care is good, satisfaction with the physical environment will be a bonus. If the patient is pleased with clinical and interpersonal care, deficiencies in the physical environment are unlikely to lead to overall dissatisfaction and the registration of a complaint.

If there is dissatisfaction with the clinical outcome or interpersonal care, a high-quality physical environment is unlikely to compensate for deficiencies in these more important aspects of care. Furthermore, a low-quality environment may provide a focus for the discontent of a patient or their relatives if there is dissatisfaction with other aspects of care that are difficult to articulate.

6.5.1.3   Interpersonal care: expectations and experience

Frank rudeness in carers is an obvious cause of dissatisfaction in patients. However, it is more common for failures in a professional's behaviour to be of a subtle non-verbal nature. It is important that any patient receives the impression that s/he:

- is an individual and not just a number;
- has a problem which is of great importance;
- is the sole focus of that professional's attention at that particular moment.

A professional may believe in this approach, but if this belief is not translated into appropriate behaviour the patient is not able to appreciate it: patients are not mind readers.

6.5.1.4   Is the measurement of patient satisfaction of any use?

The measurement of patient satisfaction is not completely pointless. One objective of any manager should be to satisfy the patient's desire for safe and effective treatment, delivered by professionals who care about that patient, in pleasant surroundings.

6.5.2   Searching

As patient satisfaction is determined to such a great extent by the local characteristics of a particular service, as opposed to its effectiveness, studies of patient satisfaction may not be considered to be research and, as such, may not be indexed in MEDLINE or EMBASE. It is still worth searching both databases using 'satisfaction' and 'patient's perception of outcome' as keywords.

6.5.3 Appraisal

Critical skills are needed for two tasks.

1. The appraisal of an instrument for measuring satisfaction. There are many such instruments, usually a combination of a questionnaire and an interview, either face to face or by telephone. A checklist of questions for the appraisal of any instrument used to assess patient satisfaction is shown in Box 6.9.
2. The appraisal of the study of patient satisfaction. Although the main focus of the appraisal is on the instrument used to measure satisfaction, it is also important to assess the overall study design (see Box 6.10).

6.5.4 Applicability and relevance

Surveys of patient satisfaction are primarily of use to the service in which they have been conducted. The degree to which any of the results are a function of patient expectations, which vary from one population to another, and the quality of the service those patients received make it difficult for findings about one service to be applied to

---

Box 6.9 Checklist for the appraisal of instruments used to assess patient satisfaction

1. How has the instrument been tested?
2. What is the interobserver variability, i.e. how different are the answers if different people use the questionnaire on the same person?
3. How good is the instrument at measuring the three aspects of care that determine satisfaction: interpersonal care, the physical environment and clinical outcome?
4. How comprehensible are the questions to people of different reading abilities or different ethnic backgrounds?

Box 6.10 Checklist for the appraisal of study designs used to assess patient satisfaction

1. How well did the survey assess the experience of the patients as opposed to their reaction to that experience?
2. Was the sample interviewed a representative sample of the population served by the service or was it biased?
3. Are the results applicable to the population in general?
4. Are the results relevant to the 'local' population?

others elsewhere. However, the reasons for complaint uncovered in such surveys (e.g. noise), as opposed to the degree of patient dissatisfaction, may be useful because they can indicate causes of dissatisfaction that could be relevant in any population.

6.5.5 Evidence-based 'friendliness'

In future, it may become equally important to use measures of clinicians' perceptions of the process of care as it becomes more difficult to recruit and retain these professionals.

A striking but little known trial is known as the 'friendly' dentists trial.[3] In this trial, two approaches to dental practice for people who required dentures were investigated: in the treatment group, the dentists discussed care options with patients, involved them in decision making and shared both the responsibility and pleasure of a satisfactory outcome; the control group received treatment in the usual manner. The outcome of the trial demonstrated clearly that the 'friendly' dentists achieved better clinical outcomes than the conventional dentists.

Evidence of the effectiveness of patient participation in the process of care was also produced by a cross-sectional survey of 7730 patients from the practices of 300 physicians.[4] In this study, which was part of the Medical Outcomes Study, it was found that:

* the greater the level of patient participation, the greater the degree of patient satisfaction;
* physicians who had primary care training or training in interviewing scored higher than those without such training;
* physicians in higher volume practices were rated as less participatory than those in lower volume practices;
* physicians who were satisfied with the level of professional autonomy were rated as more participatory than those who were dissatisfied.

The authors raise the fascinating possibility that:

'Because participatory decision-making style is related to patient satisfaction and loyalty to the physician, cost-containment strategies that reduce time with patients and decrease physician autonomy may result in suboptimal patient outcomes'.

It must be remembered that this survey was conducted within the US healthcare system, and the questionnaire had also been developed in the USA, so the results cannot be taken at face value. However, there appears to be strong evidence that a participatory, 'friendly' style of practice is better for patient care and, if patients can vote with their feet, for business.

The message: longer, 'friendlier' consultations involving greater patient participation are cost-effective in the long term, although the costs may be greater in the short term.

An editorial, entitled 'The physician interviewer in the era of corporatization of care',[5] opened with the challenging option of Sisyphus:

> 'With the increasing corporatization of medicine, are physicians becoming Sisyphean drudges toiling futilely, forced to roll the stone uphill faster and faster, losing patients, pride in quality care, autonomy, and their own health? This increasingly prevalent self-image – correlated with high rates of burnout and fundamental dissatisfaction with the profession – contrasts with the happier, Pegasus-like myth of the physician soaring on the wings of science and professionalism, experiencing the joys of effectiveness, altruism, moral probity, and wealth that attracted so many of us to medicine. Implicit in much Sisyphean negativism is victimization – by the nature of things, in Camus' existentialist version, and by the medical-industrial complex, in others. The extent to which we have perpetuated our own victimization and the extent to which it is remediable through our own actions are empiric questions.'

The author of the editorial concluded by arguing that improving interview skills improves both the physician's and the patient's satisfaction with care, and as professionals perform about 200 000–300 000 consultations in a lifetime, they can improve performance and feel better. Thus, the development of better interviewing skills should not be seen simply as an altruistic device to improve patient satisfaction, but as part of a self-interested campaign for physician survival.

References

1. CLEARY, P.D., EDGMAN-LEVITAN, S., WALKER, J.D. et al. (1993) *Using patient reports to improve medical care: a preliminary report from 10 hospitals*. Qual. Manage. Health Care 2: 31–8.
2. BRUSTER, S., JARMAN, B., BOSANQUET, N. et al. (1994) *National survey of hospital patients*. Br. Med. J. 309: 1542–6.
3. LEFER, L., PLEASURE, M.A. and RESENTHAL, L. (1962) *A psychiatric approach to the denture patient*. J. Psychosom. Res. 6: 199–207.
4. KAPLAN, S.H., GREENFIELD, S., GANDEK, B. et al. (1996) *Characteristics of physicians with participatory decision-making styles*. Ann. Intern. Med. 124: 497–504.
5. LIPKIN, M. Jr. (1996) *Sisyphus or Pegasus? The physician interviewer in the era of corporatization of care*. Ann. Intern. Med. 124: 511–2.

6.6 COST-EFFECTIVENESS

> **Oxymoron**: 'a rhetorical figure by which contradictory terms are conjoined so as to give point to the statement or expression (now often loosely = a contradiction in terms)'
>
> *Shorter Oxford English Dictionary*

The arguments used by the pharmaceutical companies have changed recently; no longer do they claim that a new drug is more effective, they emphasise that the drug is much more cost-effective for the health service, the argument being that even though the cost of prescribed medication is more expensive, savings are made elsewhere in the healthcare system.

Robert Evans, one of the world's leading health economists, has responded trenchantly to two letters in the *Annals of Internal Medicine*[1] in which a leader he wrote nine months previously was criticised. His leader,[2] which should be read by anyone who receives information about the cost-effectiveness of new drugs, was written as a commentary and critique of a major report on the principles of 'Economic Analysis of Health Care Technology'.[3] Evans pointed out that the work of the Taskforce described in the report was funded entirely by the pharmaceutical industry and that the industry was giving a verisimilitude of objectivity to a technique that should be assumed to be biased. His criticisms are typically forthright; for example, he states that:

> 'A pseudodiscipline, "pharmaco-economics", has been conjured into existence by the magic of money, with its own practitioners, conferences, and journals. There are a lot of drugs and there is a lot of money, so the "field" is booming'.

In response to the critical letters,[1] he concludes:

> 'In the end, drug buyers and reimbursers will have to do their own evaluations and make their own purchasing decisions. Offers of participation and scientific cooperation from sellers always spring from the same underlying motive, to move the product. What else can they do?'

This may seem a pessimistic line to take but this issue must be faced, especially as studies of cost-effectiveness have an increasingly important role to play in the appraisal of new interventions.

A similar line of argument was taken in a leader published in the *British Medical Journal* on 'Promoting cost-effective prescribing'.[4] It was pointed out that drug companies and those working for funders of health services can be criticised for being inevitably biased. The authors called for clear and rigorous guidelines on cost-effectiveness to be drawn up by the UK Department of Health and the Association of British Pharmaceutical Industries, and for those guidelines to be used as a 'fourth hurdle' once efficacy has been demonstrated by randomised trials, as is the case in Australia.

6.6.1   Dimensions and definitions

6.6.1.1   Efficiency and productivity

Wittgenstein proposed that when a word caused more confusion than clarification its use should be discontinued; this is surely the case with the word 'efficiency'. The term is often used synonymously with productivity. It is common in the NHS for efficiency to be calculated by relating the outputs of the service, that is, episodes of care, to the inputs, that is, costs:

$$\frac{\text{Episodes of care}}{\text{Finance}}$$

Although this is not an unreasonable definition (indeed, Cochrane used a similar definition in his excellent work *Effectiveness and Efficiency*[5]), it is a definition of productivity. Several other definitions of efficiency have been proposed;[6] for example:

$$\frac{\text{Number of episodes of care}}{\text{Number of professionals}}$$

A further example would be the number of operations per surgeon. However, these examples of the definition of 'efficiency', in which outputs are related to inputs, are in fact measures of productivity.

Cochrane's use of the term 'efficiency', although superficially similar to its present use (he cites, for example, 'length of stay' as one measure), encompasses one important difference: he focused on *effective* interventions. For Cochrane, the provision of a service of proven ineffectiveness, or of unproven efficacy, was inefficient *ipso facto* no matter how cheaply that intervention was delivered. His use of the term 'efficiency' is therefore closer to the term 'cost-effectiveness':

$$\frac{\text{Number of interventions for which there is strong evidence that they do more good than harm}}{\text{Cost}}$$

In this context, 'strong' means based on good-quality research, using the criteria set out in Chapter 5. Cost-effectiveness may be written more simply as:

$$\frac{\text{Interventions of proven effectiveness}}{\text{Cost}}$$

6.6.1.2 Using outcomes to assess efficiency

A correct measure of efficiency is to use outcomes as the numerators:

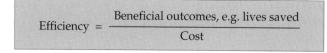

$$\text{Efficiency} = \frac{\text{Beneficial outcomes, e.g. lives saved}}{\text{Cost}}$$

If cost-effectiveness is being measured, it is essential to remember that the effects of care may be adverse as well as beneficial and the equation should read:

$$\frac{\text{Beneficial outcomes } - \text{ adverse outcomes}}{\text{Cost}}$$

The beneficial outcome of an intervention designed to prevent mortality was initially expressed only in terms of the number of extra years of life resulting from that intervention. Subsequently, it was recognised that the quality of that life is also important. Studies were undertaken to ascertain the values people attach to different states of health and illness. A method was developed that enabled a combination of a patient's levels of disability and distress, such as pain, to be assessed.[7] It was found that it was possible to reach a consensus on the value that people attached to certain states ranging from 1 which represents excellent health to 0 which represents the worst state of health. Thus, it is possible to construct the following equation:

> The number of extra years of life obtained
>
> ×
>
> The value of the quality of life
>
> =
>
> Quality Adjusted Life Years (QALYs)

6.6.1.3   Marginal and opportunity costs

To determine the cost of an operation, the cost of a unit, including all fixed costs, is divided by the number of operations performed by that unit.

$$\frac{\text{\textit{Total} cost of the unit, including salaries and capital charges (£10 000 000)}}{\text{Number of operations (1000)}} = £10\ 000$$

A marginal cost is the cost of any additional interventions performed by a unit for which the cost of working at a particular rate has already been calculated. For instance, in a unit in which 1 000 operations are undertaken at a cost of

£10 000 each, the fixed costs will be £9000 per operation whereas the cost of the consumables per operation will be £1000. Thus, the marginal cost of 100 extra operations will be £100 000, i.e. the cost of the consumables at £1000 for each operation.

Opportunity costs are defined as the other uses on which the same amount of money can be spent. For example, the opportunity costs of the £100 000 that might be spent on 100 more cardiac operations can be expressed as the number of chiropody treatments or cataract operations that could be purchased with that same amount of money.

6.6.1.4 Economic evaluations in research

There are many different approaches to the evaluation of efficiency, but those of most use to decision makers are cost–benefit analysis and cost-effectiveness analysis.

Cost–benefit analysis and cost–utility analysis enable an assessment to be made of the benefit that will be gained from investing resources in a particular type of health service. For example, the results would allow the returns on an investment in an immunisation programme to be compared with the returns that might be obtained from an investment in another child health programme, another preventive programme or any other form of healthcare.

- Cost–benefit analysis provides an assessment of the return on investment in terms of money.
- Cost–utility analysis provides an assessment of the return on investment in terms of QALYs.

Cost–benefit and cost–utility analyses enable decision makers to compare the returns on investing resources in services designed to treat different health problems, whereas studies of cost-effectiveness enable decision makers to compare the costs of different ways of tackling the same health problem.

- The results of a cost–benefit analysis would help a decision maker assess the returns on investing £100 000 additional resources in either a renal transplantation programme or a cardiac surgery programme.
- The results of a cost-effectiveness analysis would help the decision maker assess the relative cost-effectiveness of dialysis and of transplantation as methods of treating end-stage renal failure.

6.6.2 Searching

Step 1. Specify the search term for the health problem and the intervention.

Step 2. Search for terms that will identify papers focusing on the costs of the particular health problem and the cost-effectiveness of the intervention.

6.6.3 Appraisal

A checklist of questions for the appraisal of economic evaluations is shown in Box 6.11.

6.6.4 Applicability and relevance

The main problem with cost–benefit and cost-effectiveness studies is their limited relevance to decision makers responsible for populations other than those in which the study was performed.

The effectiveness of a service is universal; a service's cost-effectiveness is influenced by local factors. A cost–benefit study of a coronary artery disease programme is a function

---

Box 6.11 Checklist for the appraisal of economic evaluations of healthcare (Source: Drummond et al[6])

1. Was a well-defined question posed in an answerable form?
2. Was a comprehensive description of the competing alternatives given, i.e. is it possible to identify who did what to whom, where and how often?
3. Was there evidence that the programme's effectiveness had been established? Was this done through a randomised, controlled clinical trial? If not, how strong was the evidence of effectiveness?
4. Were all important and relevant costs and consequences for each alternative identified?
5. Were costs and consequences measured accurately in appropriate physical units (e.g. hours of nursing time, number of physician visits, days lost from work or years of life gained) prior to valuation?
6. Were costs and consequences valued credibly?
7. Were costs and consequences adjusted for differential timing?
8. Was an incremental analysis of the costs and consequences of alternatives performed? Were the additional (incremental) costs generated by the use of one alternative over another compared with the additional effects, benefits or utilities generated?
9. Was a sensitivity analysis performed?
10. Did the presentation and discussion of the results of the study include all of the issues that are of concern to users?

---

of the incidence and prevalence of coronary artery disease in the population served. Similarly, if the opportunity costs are expressed in terms of tuberculosis control they are influenced by the incidence of tuberculosis in that population.

In assessing whether any economic appraisal is relevant, it is necessary to ask:

- how similar is the population to the 'local' population?
- how similar are the healthcare costs to 'local' costs?

Data showing the relative costs and benefits of different programmes are more useful than absolute data about one programme, but the results of all economic studies must be used with caution.

References

1. EVANS, R.G. (1996) *Principles of economic analysis of health care technology. [Response to letters]* Ann. Intern. Med. 124: 536.
2. EVANS, R.G. (1995) *Manufacturing consensus, marketing truth: guidelines for economic evaluation.* Ann. Intern. Med. 123: 59–60.
3. TASK FORCE ON PRINCIPLES FOR ECONOMIC ANALYSIS OF HEALTH CARE TECHNOLOGY (1995) *Economic analysis of health care technology. A report on principles.* Ann. Intern. Med. 123: 61–70.
4. FREEMANTLE, N., HENRY, D., MAYNARD, A. and TORRANCE, G. (1995) *Promoting cost-effective prescribing.* Br. Med. J. 310: 955–6.
5. COCHRANE, A. (1972) *Effectiveness and Efficiency.* Nuffield Provincial Hospitals Trust, London.
6. DRUMMOND, M.F., STODDART, G.L. and TORRANCE, G.A. (1987) *Methods for the Economic Evaluation of Health Care Programmes.* Oxford University Press, Oxford.
7. ROSSER, R. and KIND, P. (1978) *A scale of valuations of states of illness: is there a sound consensus?* Int. J. Epidemiol. 7: 347–58.

6.7 QUALITY

Arguments about the relative superiority of process measures and outcome measures in the assessment of quality have been waged since the concepts were first introduced by Avedis Donabedian. The process of care is the healthcare activity or set of activities undertaken from admission of a patient to hospital or on operation; the outcome of care is the result of undertaking those activities.

When outcome measures were first proposed they were hailed as the ultimate measures that would enable the patient and purchaser to distinguish a good service from a bad service. Further experience with outcome-based measures of quality dimmed this initial enthusiasm for two main reasons.[1]

1. The health status of an individual, a group of patients or a population receiving a service is determined by several factors other than the quality of that service, notably, severity of illness and state of health before treatment.
2. The collection of valid information about outcomes in ordinary service settings is difficult because of the problems of obtaining accurate information on the presence of other complicating diseases.

Thus, although both process and outcome measures can be used in the assessment of quality, process measures are better.

6.7.1 Dimensions and definitions

6.7.1.1 Quality assessment by measuring the process of care

The effectiveness of a professional or a service is the degree to which the objectives of care are achieved, whereas the quality of a service is the degree to which it conforms to preset standards of care.

A standard is developed as part of a system of care, that system comprising a set of activities which have common objectives. The objectives for any service should be expressed in terms of the population served whenever possible, as the objectives for the NHS Breast Screening Programme demonstrate (see Box 6.12).

In a cervical screening programme, although mortality rates from cervical cancer are the only measures those responsible for national policy should use, for those responsible for 'local' services this outcome measure is not a good indicator of service quality for two reasons.

1. Changes in mortality rates are influenced by factors other than service quality, for example, changes in the incidence of cervical cancer.
2. Changes in mortality rate reflect the quality of the service pertaining several years ago, whereas the manager or purchaser needs information about the current state of quality.

Outcomes are rarely of use in measuring quality. For each objective for any service, relevant healthcare activities need to be identified, the rates of delivery of which can be used to measure progress towards the objective. The healthcare activities chosen to indicate the rate of progress towards an objective were called process measures by Donabedian.[2]

Box 6.12   Original objectives of the NHS Breast Screening Programme

The aim of the programme is to reduce mortality from breast cancer in the population screened.

- To identify and invite eligible women for mammographic screening.
- To carry out mammography in a high proportion of those who were invited.
- To provide services that are acceptable to those who receive them.
- To follow up all women referred for further investigations.
- To minimise the adverse effects of screening – anxiety, radiation and unnecessary investigations.
- To diagnose cancers accurately.
- To support and carry out research.
- To make effective and efficient use of resources for the benefit of the whole population.
- To enable those working in the programme to develop their skills and find fulfilment in their work.
- To encourage the provision of effective acceptable treatment which has minimal psychological or functional side-effects.
- To evaluate the service regularly and provide feedback to the population served.

The processes measured should be those for which there is good evidence of effectiveness. For example, for an assessment of the quality of a maternity service, the proportion of women going into labour prematurely who were given antenatal steroids[3] is an evidence-based process measure; in the assessment of the quality of care received by those with acute myocardial infarction, the proportion of patients who receive streptokinase treatment within an hour of arriving at hospital is also an evidence-based process measure.

By using these evidence-based process measures, the performance of an individual or service can be defined; this is an objective assessment of what *is* being achieved. A standard is a subjective judgement of a level of performance that *could* be achieved.

Different types of standard can be set.

- The minimal acceptable standard below which no service should fall without urgent remedial action being taken.
- The optimal standard: the best level of service that can be achieved. Although this is a worthy standard, it is often achieved only by exceptional people and/or people working in exceptional circumstances. The optimal

standard may be regarded by colleagues in other services as atypical and therefore of little use for motivating the majority of service providers.

- The achievable standard: the level of performance achieved by the top quartile of services; if one quartile of services can achieve a certain performance level, almost all services have the potential to do so.

A comparison of actual performance with the standard enables a target for quality improvement to be set. These elements can be combined into a system of care shown in Fig. 6.4.

6.7.1.2 Quality assessment by measuring the outcome of care

Although it has not proved possible to collect information on outcomes for subsequent utilisation in large databases of sufficiently good quality to allow the adequate evaluation of new interventions, there is still hope that such databases can be used to provide useful information on the quality of services delivered by either institutions or clinicians. Outcome measures, e.g. mortality rates for patients with specific conditions such as myocardial infarction, are now being used in 'league tables' of hospital quality. However, numerous practical problems have to be resolved to ensure that databases hold accurate data on each and every case treated within a service; unless there is complete coverage, any conclusions drawn from an analysis of such databases may be misleading. Furthermore, completeness of data

| Objectives | Criteria | Standards | | Present position | Targets |
		Minimal	Achievable		
To cover the population who would benefit from cervical screening	Percentage of women who have **not** had a hysterectomy who have had a readable smear in the last 5 years	50%	80%	70 general practices under 50%	By the end of year: 1 out of 70 general practices less than 50%
				17 practices more than 80%	35 general practices over 80%

Fig. 6.4

(in terms of quantity and quality) for all cases does not resolve all of the problems because, in any comparison, factors such as co-morbidity and disease severity must be taken into account.

'Co-morbidity' is the presence of other conditions that may be relevant to a patient's outcome; 'severity' describes the stage of disease a patient has. Those hospitals in which there are selective admission procedures, i.e. certain patients who have significant co-morbidity or a severe form of a disease are excluded, may appear to have better outcome figures than those hospitals in which either all patients are admitted or more difficult cases are treated. Indeed, the standard of care at hospitals with selective admission procedures may be no better, it may even be worse, than that in a hospital to which all cases are admitted. Failure to correct for co-morbidity and/or disease severity is the most common reason why false conclusions are drawn from such databases. Any league tables generated from databases for which co-morbidity and disease severity data are not routinely collected are of limited credibility, particularly to those hospitals at which performance appears to be poor.

The benefits and hazards of reporting medical outcomes in the public domain are set out in an excellent article[4] describing the work done by the New York (NY) State Department of Health to reduce mortality after coronary artery bypass grafting (CABG). In 1989, the NY State Cardiac Advisory Committee helped the NY Department of Health to set up a Cardiac Surgery Reporting System to collect information about demographic variables, risk factors and complications, and about mortality after operation. In 1990, the Department published the risk-adjusted mortality rates for each hospital. Using the Freedom of Information Law, a newspaper sued the Department to obtain the basic data from which these rates had been calculated and won. The base data were published in December 1991 to a stormy reaction from the participating surgeons. Despite this, the NY Department of Health continued with the programme.

An analysis of the data showed that from the beginning of 1989 through to the end of 1992 there was a 41% decline in risk-adjusted operative mortality. No comparable data exist, and many factors could explain this decline in mortality, but it is reasonable to assume that the reporting system was responsible for part of the improvement seen.

The improvement may have resulted from the ability to identify surgeons who had poor records, usually those performing only a small number of procedures: between 1989 and 1992, 27 low-volume surgeons stopped performing CABG in New York State. Although this programme was bold and scientifically rigorous, it should be possible to use this approach elsewhere to improve performance for specific procedures which are relatively few in number but which have dramatic outcomes (e.g. death). It is not unrealistic to pursue an objective of making hospital- and operator-specific information publicly available for a small number of interventions.

6.7.2 Searching for and appraising evidence on standards of care

6.7.2.1 Searching for papers on quality standards

Step 1. Specify the intervention.

Step 2. Select terms to define the parameters that are relevant:

- quality;
- audit;
- standards.

6.7.2.2 Appraising evidence on quality standards

The most appropriate form of study design is one in which a service is followed over a period of time, not only to measure performance against agreed quality standards but also to assess the effects of the interventions designed to improve quality by measuring performance on at least two separate occasions. A checklist of questions for the appraisal of evidence on quality is shown in Box 6.13.

Box 6.13 Checklist for the appraisal of evidence on quality

1. Is there good evidence that the intervention used as the indicator of quality is an effective intervention?
2. Are there standards relating to acceptability and safety?
3. Is there clear information about the method used to develop the standards, e.g. are the standards set by taking the cut-off point for the top quartile of several services?
4. Is there only one measure of quality or are there several measures?

6.7.3   Searching for and appraising evidence on variations in healthcare outcome

The search for and appraisal of evidence setting out standards of care and means of quality improvement is often driven by the professionals or managers within a service. However, external forces, such as the publication of interhospital audit results or hospital mortality league tables, may raise the issue. Although poor performance may stimulate only denial, a more scientific approach is possible.

6.7.3.1   Searching for papers on variations in healthcare outcome

Step 1.   Take the disease or health problem and explode the term.

Step 2.   Combine the search results with the name of the operation and/or with the term 'mortality'. It may be necessary to explode 'mortality'.

6.7.3.2   Appraising evidence on variations in healthcare outcome

Large databases can also be manipulated to compare different types of institution, for example:

- teaching hospitals *vs* non-teaching hospitals;
- services providing a high volume of care *vs* those providing a low volume.

For this type of comparison, it is not possible to perform an RCT; however, the 'natural experiment' created by the variety of health services provides an opportunity to identify the determinants of quality.

A checklist of questions for the appraisal of studies designed to investigate a possible managerial problem or to identify the determinants of service quality is shown in Box 6.14.

6.7.4   Applicability and relevance

Is it possible to apply the results of studies on quality of care from one organisation or population to another? It has been argued that because health services and methods of payment vary greatly from one population to another work on quality is not generalisable and is specific to the population in which the study was done.

Box 6.14 Checklist for the appraisal of studies of quality in the provision of healthcare (Source: Adapted from Naylor and Guyatt[5])

1. Are the outcome measures accurate and comprehensive?
   Large databases tend to include only simple outcome measures, such as death, and rarely hold data on measures such as disability or quality of life.

2. Were there clearly identified and appropriate comparison groups?
   The groups compared may simply be the two groups of patients within the two types of hospital under investigation, but a better technique is to use the standardised mortality ratios (SMRs) of all people of the same age as the two groups being studied as the yardstick against which the mortality of both groups can be measured.[6]

3. Were the comparison groups similar with respect to important determinants of outcome other than the one of interest?
   For example, when comparing teaching hospitals with non-teaching hospitals, the question must be asked: 'Are the two groups of patients similar from the point of view, for example, of the prognosis?'.

   Useful appraisal questions to ask include:

   - Did the investigators measure all known important prognostic factors?
   - Were measures of patients' prognostic factors reproducible and accurate?
   - Did the investigators show the extent to which patients differ on these factors?
   - Did the researchers use some form of multivariate analysis to adjust for all the important prognostic factors?
   - Did additional analysis (particularly in low-risk subgroups) demonstrate the same results as the primary analysis?

4. Were all possible hypotheses examined?
   Often the report of an observational study has as a focus the most dramatic finding, e.g. a difference between teaching and non-teaching hospitals, but when comparing services in which there are differences in the same outcome measure more than one explanation is possible.

   - Who did the operation, e.g. specialist or generalist?
     - When was it done, e.g. day or night, weekday or weekend?
     - Where was it done, e.g. in a large-volume or small-volume service?
     - How was it done?
     - Which operation was done?

It is true that the *results* of studies of quality are not generalisable: poor quality of care in a service such as cervical screening in one population does not mean that the quality of cervical screening will be poor in all populations. However, the identification of criteria that can be used to set standards and measure quality and of the reasons for quality failure are generalisable. For example, in the study of CABG in New York State,[4] the identification of the high risk of mortality associated with low-volume surgeons is a generalisable finding. It is immaterial whether the high mortality rate was because those surgeons were less practised in the operation or fewer patients were referred to those surgeons because referring physicians were aware of their performance (a common quality standard used within the profession), the association was demonstrated and is relevant to all parties – patients, physicians, providers and purchasers.

References

1. SCHROEDER, S. A., and KABCENELL, A. I. (1991) *Do bad outcomes mean substandard care?* JAMA 265: 1995.
2. DONABEDIAN, A. (1980) *The definition of quality: a conceptual exploration.* In *Explorations in Quality Assessment and Monitoring. Volume I: The Definition of Quality and Approaches to Its Assessment.* Health Administration Press, Ann Arbor.
3. CROWLEY, P.A. et al. (1995) *Antenatal corticosteroid therapy: a meta-analysis of the randomized trials, 1972 to 1994.* Am. J. Obstet. Gynecol. 173: 322–5.
4. CHASSIN, M.R., HANNAN, R.L. and DeBUONO, B.A. (1996) *Benefits and hazards of reporting medical outcomes publicly.* New Eng. J. Med. 334: 394-8.
5. NAYLOR, C.D. and GUYATT, G.H. (1996) *User's Guides to the Medical Literature. X. How to use an article reporting variations in the outcomes of health services.* JAMA 275: 554–8.
6. SEAGROATT, V. and GOLDACRE, M.J. (1994) *Measures of early postoperative mortality beyond hospital fatality rates.* Br. Med. J. 309: 361–5.

6.8 APPROPRIATENESS

6.8.1 Dimensions and definitions

The effectiveness of an intervention is the degree to which the objectives governing its use have been achieved. Appropriateness is a measure of the use of the intervention and is a subjective judgement based on a balance of probabilities: the probability of doing good against the probability of doing harm.

A study of appropriateness is designed to reveal whether the right patient is given the right treatment at the right time by the right professional in the right place.

In clinical practice, any judgement of appropriateness should take into account the needs, values and expressed wishes of the individual patient. Chemotherapy with agents that carry a high probability of side-effects may be appropriate for a patient with potentially curable cancer but may be inappropriate for a patient who has incurable cancer, depending upon the relative values that patient attaches to a few more months of life on the one hand and to suffering side-effects on the other.

The concept of appropriateness is particularly useful when making decisions about what Naylor has called the 'grey zones of clinical practice', namely, aspects of care for which the evidence is scarce or the evidence available is not relevant to the patients or the service under consideration.[1]

Hitherto, financial cost has not been a factor in clinical decisions about appropriateness relating to individual patients, but for populations the concept of appropriateness relates not only to benefits and risks but also to the costs of intervention. Furthermore, the appropriateness of an intervention or a service for any population may change with the volume of service provided. If resources are limited, a service is usually given to those who are most likely to benefit. As resources increase, the threshold for intervention changes and the intervention is offered to people who are at lower risk or less severely affected. The benefit obtained with each unit of increase in resources decreases – the law of diminishing returns – with a flattening of the cost–benefit curve (Fig. 6.5).

Interventions have adverse as well as beneficial effects. Donabedian, who invented the concept of 'structure, process and outcome' in healthcare evaluation, introduced the benefit-to-harm graph.[2] He argued that when the volume of healthcare offered is increased, the cost–benefit curve flattens but the cost–harm curve does not; namely, side-effects may be as common in individuals at low risk or who have mild disease as in those at high risk or who have severe disease. For each unit increase in resources or volume of care, there is a concomitant increase in adverse effects (Fig. 6.6).

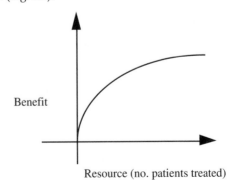

Fig. 6.5
(Source: Donabedian; see ref. 2, p. 147)

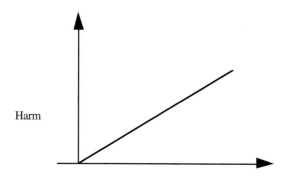

Harm

Resource (no. patients treated)

Fig. 6.6
(Source: Donabedian; see ref. 2, p. 147)

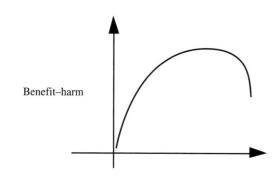

Benefit–harm

Fig. 6.7
(Source: Donabedian; see ref. 2, p. 147)

Thus, as the proportion of a population covered by a health service increases, the balance of good to harm changes. This can be expressed most simply by subtracting harm from good and showing the net benefit graphically (Fig. 6.7).

There are several ways in which the appropriateness of use of a particular intervention may be identified as a matter of concern, notably:

- as part of an audit project;
- following the publication of an article on appropriateness;
- following the publication of a league table showing variations in the rate of utilisation of a particular intervention by different clinicians or services; pressure falls on the professional or service at the end of the table deemed to be the least appropriate.

Evidence-based analysis of variations in levels of utilisation may indicate variations in appropriateness of use (remember variations in *outcome* may indicate variations in quality) (Table 6.4).

Table 6.4

Variation	Possible problem
In outcome	Quality
In rates of intervention	Appropriateness

6.8.1.1 *It may be appropriate but is it necessary?*

Once all ineffective interventions and services have been excluded, if resources are limited it may not be possible to provide all of the effective and appropriate services. The team from the RAND Health Sciences Program has developed a new criterion that can be used to evaluate appropriate interventions: necessity.[3] Their definition of appropriateness is that the benefits should sufficiently outweigh the risks to make the procedure worth performing, and they extend this definition by proposing criteria that can be used to decide whether a procedure is necessary or crucial (see Box 6.15).

A high necessity rating indicates that it is improper clinical judgement not to recommend the procedure; a low necessity rating indicates that there are alternative courses of action (including no action) that are equally or almost equally appropriate. This is an important and novel way of thinking about procedures and is already being used by the RAND team.

Box 6.15   Criteria for identifying necessary or crucial interventions (all four must be met) (Source: Kahan et al[3])

- The procedure must be *appropriate,* as defined above.
- It would be improper care not to recommend this service.
- There is a reasonable chance that the procedure will benefit the patient. Procedures with a low likelihood of benefit but few risks are not considered necessary.
- The benefit to the patient is not small. Procedures that provide only minor benefits are not necessary.

Necessity can be measured by asking a panel of clinicians to rate a set of cases. Although there is, as would be expected, variation in rating, there is sufficient consistency for the measure of necessity to be useful. One obvious use is to determine which procedures are not necessary to the well-being of patients. However, the RAND team points out that the converse is also possible, namely, that patients do not receive necessary treatment either because of costs or because of the judgement of the clinicians. The RAND team reviewed 243 patients with angina who had positive exercise stress tests. They found that patients who were under the care of a cardiologist were more likely to receive a 'necessary' exercise stress test than those who were under the care of a generalist or primary care physician.[4]

6.8.2   Searching

Step 1. Specify the intervention for which there are different rates of utilisation. The relevant MeSH term is 'utilization review', an American term similar to 'clinical audit'. It may be necessary to explode 'utilization review'.

Step 2. Search for 'guideline' or 'practice guideline' under publication type.

Step 3. The relevant MeSH term is 'guidelines'; the term should be exploded to include 'practice guidelines'.

Step 4. The keywords 'guideline' and 'appropriateness' can be used. The MeSH term for appropriateness is 'regional health planning', which it may be necessary to explode.

6.8.3   Appraisal

Most of the research published on appropriateness is a review of data about patients that were collected previously. A checklist of three sets of questions useful for the appraisal of evidence of appropriateness is shown in Box 6.16.

> **Box 6.16** Checklist for the appraisal of evidence of appropriateness
> (Source: Adapted from Naylor and Guyatt[5])
>
> 1. Are the criteria evidence based?
>   - Is there evidence to support the judgements about:
>   - right patient?
>   - right place?
>   - right time?
>   - right intervention?
>   - right professional?
>   - What is the quality of the evidence on which the judgements have been made and the criteria chosen?
>   - How good was the agreement between experts on the panel?
>   - Were patients' views on outcomes taken into account?
>
> 2. How scientifically was the study done?
>   - Were steps taken to minimise bias, for example, by using more than one auditor or by using explicit criteria to audit notes?
>   - Was the sample of patients representative and large enough to produce valid results?
>
> 3. Are the criteria relevant to the 'local' service?
>   - How similar is the 'local' population to the population studied?
>   - Were the clinicians on the panel similar to 'local' professionals?
>   - How different from the 'local' facility was the facility studied?

6.8.4 Applicability and relevance

Appropriateness is a subjective measure of whether an intervention, or level of intervention, is right; this judgement of 'rightness' is influenced by the incidence or prevalence of the disease in the population and by the resources available.

Although the results of studies of appropriateness may not be generalisable, they may be of relevance to different populations because they can reveal areas of clinical uncertainty. Thus, a study of appropriateness could indicate an interesting area to investigate in the 'local' health service; if validated, the methods used in the study can probably be transposed, with modification. However, the levels of intervention judged to be 'right' for the 'local' population must be determined according to 'local' circumstances.

References

1. NAYLOR, C.D. (1995) *The grey zones of clinical practice.* Lancet 345: 840–2.
2. DONABEDIAN, A. (1980) *Explorations in Quality Assessment and Monitoring. Volume 1: The Definition of Quality and Approaches to Its Assessment.* Health Administration Press, Ann Arbor.
3. KAHAN, J.P., BERNSTEIN, S.J., LEAPE, L.L. et al. (1994) *Measuring the necessity of medical procedures.* Med. Care 32: 357–65.
4. BOROWSKY, S.J., KRAVITZ, R.L., LAOURI, M. et al. (1995) *Effect of physician specialty on use of necessary coronary angiography.* J. Am. Coll. Cardiol. 26: 1484–91.
5. NAYLOR, C.D. and GUYATT, G.H. (1996) *User's Guides to the Medical Literature. XI. How to use an article about a clinical utilization review.* JAMA 275: 1435–40.

PROLOGUE 7

Dear Reader,

Empathise with the Secretary of the Faculty of Public Health Screening Committee. He was musing on the particular lightness of green which makes the leaves of early summer stand out sharply against the blue sky of May. The movement of the leaves was a comfort to him. He looked at them for at least three minutes before letting his eyes drop to the letter, written in innocence but devastating in its content, which lay on the desk before him.

'Dear Colleague, I would be grateful to know the evidence to support the introduction of screening for abdominal aortic aneurysm which we are currently considering.
The proposal is strongly supported.
It would have a very beneficial impact on our efficiency index because many more people would be referred to hospital but I would also be interested to know what health benefits we can describe to the health authority.'

Commentary

Organisations take on a life of their own. The culture of an organisation imbues any decision making with the prevailing preoccupation, in this case a preoccupation with productivity. To counteract this, a different hierarchy within the decision-making process is vital, one in which it is possible to ask the following questions.

- *Will the proposal have a beneficial effect on health?*
- *Is there a harmful effect, and what is the balance between benefit and harm?*
- *What is the cost of the innovation?*
- *How does this proposal compare with other proposals currently under consideration?*
- *Is it possible to deliver the new service at acceptable levels of quality and cost?*

CHAPTER 7

ORGANISATIONAL DEVELOPMENT FOR EVIDENCE-BASED HEALTHCARE

A health service consists of:

- organisations, i.e. a set of units and individuals who work together;
- systems of care through which patients travel, a system being a series of functions which have a common set of objectives;
- clinical encounters, during which clinicians and patients make decisions that can alter a patient's course through that system and improve their health (Chapter 9).

7.1 KEY COMPONENTS OF AN EVIDENCE-BASED HEALTH SERVICE

The key components in an evidence-based service are:

1. organisations designed with the capability to generate and the flexibility to incorporate evidence;
2. individuals and teams who can find, appraise and use research evidence.

These two components are inter-related, as can be seen in Fig. 7.1.

For any organisation to increase the degree to which decisions taken within it are evidence based, it is important to develop the right systems and culture; it may also be necessary to change the structure of the organisation.

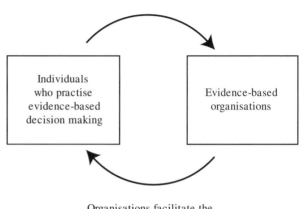

Fig. 7.1

7.1.1   The evidence-based organisation

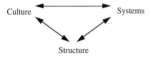

- The culture of an evidence-based organisation is an obsession with finding, appraising and using research-based knowledge in decision making.
- A system is a set of activities that have a common set of objectives. In the evidence-based organisation, in any system in which decisions are made, research-based knowledge must be sought, appraised and used as evidence when making decisions. Within the organisation there will also be a system for managing knowledge and a system for developing the skills of the individuals who work in that organisation.
- The organisation's structure should promote and facilitate evidence-based decision making.

7.1.2   The evidence-based chief executive

It is vital that the promotion of evidence-based decision making is not a task assigned solely to the medical director or director responsible for R&D or clinical development, although such personnel do have a central role in this activity; the chief executive must also be committed to evidence-based decision making. S/he must be able, and be seen, to:

- search for evidence, alone if necessary;
- appraise evidence, having participated in a critical appraisal skills workshop;

- store important evidence in a way that allows it to be retrieved using a computer;
- use evidence to make decisions: for example, by asking at least once a week, 'What is the evidence for this?', followed by a supplementary question about the quality of the evidence if this information is not proffered; by prefacing propositions with 'The evidence is …' if evidence is available (such propositions can be distinguished from statements prefaced by 'I think …' or 'In my opinion…' which, although valid, are subjective and therefore fall into a different category of proposition);
- help those individuals accountable to the chief executive to develop skills for using evidence and to change the systems for which they are responsible such that evidence can be incorporated into decision making.

7.1.3 Evidence-based everything

Dear Reader,

Empathise with the medical director. He ground his teeth and bit his tongue: 'The third financial ledger system being introduced in less than 5 years and there's no evidence to suggest that this system will be any better than the other two. Hundreds of thousands of pounds have been spent and no-one even asked for the evidence of effectiveness when the decisions were being made about which information systems to buy, particularly the financial information systems. All they kept banging on about was clinical effectiveness. What about some evidence-based management in this organisation?'

There has been much emphasis on the need to improve clinical effectiveness and to promote evidence-based clinical practice. In this book, the need to be more scientific and use evidence when making purchasing and managerial decisions about clinical services has been promoted, but what of the need to use evidence in managerial decisions about management? What was the strength of the evidence on which the decision to introduce resource management was based? How good is the evidence used to justify investment in new IT? This book has been focused primarily on decisions about clinical services mainly because there is a paucity of evidence on the effectiveness, or cost-effectiveness, of different management arrangements. It is important, however, to ensure that a scientific approach is taken to all aspects of the work of a health service provider because cost pressures may be generated by multiple small changes, as the example below illustrates.

> Barchester District General Hospital has 140 consultants and a turnover of £80 million – £570 000 per consultant per year. In one year, about 3 000 000 clinical decisions are made that will affect resource use. If each consultant were to change their clinical practice by increasing the volume or intensity of care at a cost of about £3000 (an increase of 0.52%), because of an increase in clinical and support costs which may not fall within their directorate, the Trust and its purchasers would face an increased cost of £420 000 a year. This would cause a major problem, yet which clinician would recognise a change of 0.52% in their practice?

7.1.4   Systems that provide evidence

The evidence-based organisation should have as an objective that evidence be found to support decisions. It should also be composed of systems that are capable of:

- providing evidence;
- promoting the use of evidence;
- consuming evidence.

7.1.4.1   The 'evidence centre'

Such an organisation needs an 'evidence centre', which has:

- access to the World Wide Web;
- subscriptions to the most relevant sources of data, such as MEDLINE and the Cochrane Database of Systematic Reviews;
- a limited number of appropriate books and journals;
- arrangements for obtaining documents or copies thereof, for example, reprints of articles;
- personnel who can manage these resources and promote their use.

The 'evidence centre' should not only be a location that decision makers can visit but also a 'resource' that can be accessed to provide evidence when it is needed. To fulfil the

Table 7.1

System	Drawback	Advantages
Walk or drive to the library	Time	Break from work
Exit from patient record computer system and access the 'evidence centre'	Time	Possible within hospitals at present; no technology required
Consult 'evidence centre' through a parallel system while patient record is still running	Expensive: two systems needed	Possible at present; needs separate telephone line for primary care
Consult evidence base on lap top or palm top	Expensive (but getting cheaper)	Portable system
Cue cards appear on screen with evidence and guidelines when diagnosis, patient's name or test result is entered	None	Minimises time and facilitates incorporation of evidence

latter function, it is important to consider not only what evidence is needed but also in what situations and in what form.

The commonest situations in which evidence will be needed are in a meeting or in a clinic. At present, most decision makers would have to walk to the library or, in the case of general practitioners, drive to the hospital, park the car (often a nightmare), then walk to the library, find the evidence and drive back to the health centre. The barriers to accessing evidence are often too great. A series of systems for accessing evidence is shown in Table 7.1.

7.1.5 Systems that promote the use of evidence

7.1.5.1 Evidence-based clinical audit

Evidence should be incorporated as an element into the audit cycle (see Fig. 7.2).

There are two ways in which this can be done:

1. ensure that the evidence of effectiveness or safety for the intervention being subject to the audit process is of good quality;
2. ensure that the standards applied within the audit process are scientific.

It is possible to select subjects for audit and suitable services for purchasing by analysing the research evidence. In the UK, the North Thames Regional Health Authority commissioned the London School of Hygiene and Tropical Medicine to undertake such an exercise; 10 topics were identified in a review of opportunities for evidence-based audit and purchasing (see Box 7.1).[1]

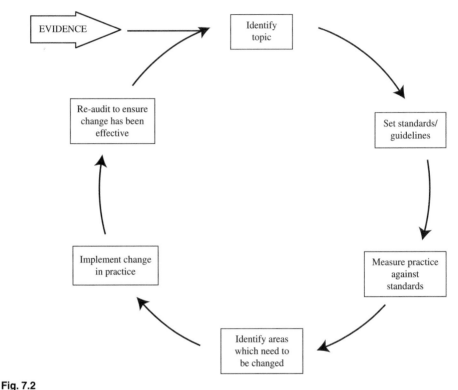

Fig. 7.2
The evidence-driven audit cycle

Box 7.1   Evidence-based opportunities for audit (Source: Sanderson[1])

1. Prenatal steroids to prevent respiratory distress syndrome
2. Vacuum extraction *vs* forceps for obstetric delivery
3. Diagnostic D&C in young women
4. Systemic adjuvant therapy for breast cancer
5. Treatment of *H. pylori* to prevent recurrence of ulcer
6. Thromboprophylaxis for orthopaedic and general surgery
7. Management of mild hypertension
8. Cholesterol screening and use of cholesterol-lowering drugs
9. Aspirin, thrombolysis and anticoagulation after myocardial infarction
10. ACE inhibitors for chronic heart failure

For each service or type of treatment, it is also possible to identify those interventions that are necessary in achieving a good outcome. This approach allows the identification of criteria that can be used to measure quality. A list of evidence-based criteria for the management of elderly patients with fractured neck of femur is shown in Box 7.2.[2–5]

Box 7.2 Evidence-based criteria for the management of elderly patients with fractured neck of femur (Source: various[2-5])

1. Spending less than one hour in casualty
2. Receiving prophylactic antibiotics
3. Receiving pharmaceutical thromboembolic prophylaxis
4. Having surgery within 24 hours
5. Recording the grade of surgeon and anaesthetist performing the operation
6. Number of days after surgery by which 50% of patients were mobilised
7. Occurrence of pressure sores, urinary tract infection and pneumonia
8. Provision of a thorough medical and social assessment
9. Degree and effectiveness of joint working between orthopaedic surgeons and consultants in medicine for the elderly
10. Adequacy of discharge planning and implementation

7.1.5.2   Training for evidence-based decision making

Within the training and development programme of any organisation, there must be strategies to develop the skills of all personnel such that they can practise evidence-based decision making and:

- search for evidence (Section 8.1);
- appraise evidence (Section 8.2);
- store evidence (Section 8.3);
- use evidence.

In the past, health service managers were responsible for organisations and systems; it was the responsibility of the professions within and the educational establishments related to the health service to influence individual clinicians. This division of responsibilities has now changed for two reasons:

1. the professions and the educational establishments are thought to have been too slow in promoting evidence-based clinical practice;
2. it has been recognised that the development of systems and of individuals are inter-related (see Fig. 7.1).

Moreover, as those who pay for and manage health services must identify the resources to invest in audit and continuing professional development, they are interested in which types of intervention are effective in bringing about change in professional practice. Although certain interventions have already been shown to be effective, more detailed work is being done, as part of the Cochrane Collaboration,[6] to review the effectiveness of the interventions shown in Box 7.3.

Box 7.3   Interventions under review for effectiveness (Source: Freemantle et al[6])

- Audit and feedback
- Printed educational materials
- Opinion leaders
- Educational outreach
- The extended role of the pharmacist
- Nursing care planning
- Computerised drug information and dosage
- Reminders and prompts
- Guidelines and protocols
- Patient penalties
- Mass media strategies
- Conferences, seminars and training attachments (preceptorships)

7.1.6   Systems that should be more evidence based

Evidence should be used to inform every decision, but there are some aspects of healthcare for which the evidence is scanty. There are, however, other aspects to which evidence could and should be applied to a much greater degree than at present, not only because evidence is available but also because its use will ensure that the best value is obtained from the resources available. Two such examples are:

- drugs and therapeutics decision making;
- equipment purchasing.

Decision making about drugs is usually centralised within a hospital or primary care team and therefore it is possible to control it; there are also good sources of information about the costs, safety and effectiveness of new drugs, which provide a sound evidence base. Decision making about the purchase of equipment is more problematic: there is less evidence available and the available evidence is of poor quality, partly because RCTs are more difficult to organise and partly because there is no requirement to demonstrate efficacy before introducing a new piece of equipment, as is the case for new drugs.

Most hospitals have an 'equipment bank' or similar budget, into which has to be incorporated some degree of equity among different departments. The consequence of this arrangement may be that a particular department requests a new piece of equipment because it is 'their turn', even if good evidence cannot be presented to support the application. As equipment budgets are limited, equipment is often bought with money raised by public subscription, for example, through a 'scanner appeal', the consequence of which is that equipment purchase often bypasses any form of evaluation (see Fig. 7.4).

A checklist of questions useful when eliciting the evidence base for any change in clinical practice is shown in Box 7.4; these questions can be applied to any proposals for the introduction of new drugs or new equipment and should be incorporated into the system in which information is collected for decision making.

For this type of appraisal to be effective when conducted on a 'local' service, it must be complemented by more exacting appraisal nationally. At present, before a drug is licensed and made available for widespread prescription, it must have been demonstrated to be efficacious and safe. In some countries, notably Australia, there is greater control over the introduction of new drugs.[7] The approach developed in Australia is set out in the Guidelines for the Pharmaceutical Industry on Preparation of Submissions to the Pharmaceutical Benefits Advisory Committee (PBAC) (see also Fig. 7.3).

Box 7.4 Checklist for the appraisal of proposals to change clinical practice

1. How did you search for evidence to support this proposal? (Please append the search strategy to this application.)
2. What is the best quality evidence supporting the proposal?
3. What will be the magnitude of the benefit compared with present practice? (Please give estimates based on the most optimistic and the most pessimistic estimate of the effect – the upper and lower confidence intervals.)
4. Compared with present practice, will there be any changes in:
   - patient safety?
   - acceptability and patient satisfaction?
   - cost:
     a) to your directorate?
     b) to any other directorate?
     c) to any other part of the health service?

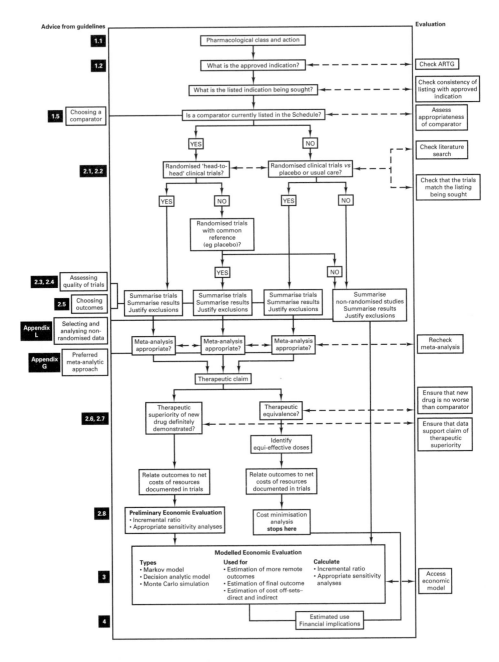

Fig. 7.3
Schema of key decisions in preparing and evaluating major submissions to the PBAC.
(Source: PBAC Guidelines)

7.1.7 Systems for managing innovation

Any issue of any journal might contain material that could prompt a clinician to make changes to their clinical practice; the issue of the *Annals of Internal Medicine* published on 15 August 1995 is taken as an example (see Box 7.5).

As can be seen from Box 7.5, there can be as many as five innovations in knowledge and technology in a single biweekly journal; extrapolating from this figure, there may be over 100 innovations a year in only one journal. Given the large number of innovations being developed and published, it is essential to institute a system whereby the introduction of any innovation is managed.

There are two types of innovation: new knowledge and new technology. At present, new technology may enter directly into the service without evaluation, whereas new knowledge does not become incorporated into clinical practice rapidly or systematically (see Fig. 7.4).

Those who purchase or provide healthcare must have systems to manage the introduction of innovation; for example, an implementation committee could be set up to decide:

- what action, if any, is needed in the light of new knowledge;
- what new technology should be introduced;
- what new technology should be prevented from entering the service, or removed from the service if it is currently being offered and yet known to be ineffective.

Box 7.5

- An RCT of a drug in which it was found to reduce gastrointestinal complications in the treatment of rheumatoid arthritis.
- A cost-effectiveness analysis of high-tech and low-tech strategies for managing suspected peptic ulcer disease.
- The use of hepatic vein insulin measurement to diagnose an insulinoma.
- A comparison of two different techniques for managing bleeding veins in the oesophagus.
- Different strategies for managing chest pain in accident and emergency, including radioisotope single photon emission computed tomographic imaging and the proposal that a cardiologist be available to see all patients suffering from chest pain.

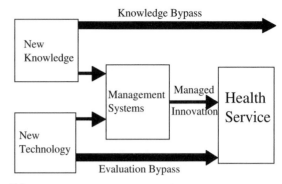

Fig. 7.4
The two main bypass routes for innovations in healthcare

7.1.8   Getting the act together

Although more resources could be spent on the promotion of evidence-based management, it is possible to make better use of the resources currently allocated to one function but assigned amongst different directorates within a hospital, such as the library, audit resources and educational resources. At some hospitals, these disparate elements are now being combined into directorates of clinical effectiveness; the checklist used in one NHS Trust is shown in Table 7.2.

Table 7.2   Clinical development directorate: activities and roles (Source: Summerton[8])

How do we find information?	Literature searching	L, CE, A
Is the information of good quality?	Validation	CE, S (A, L, M)
Is it right for the population we treat?	Applicability	CE, S (A, L, M)
How do we tell people about it?	Dissemination/education	CE, M, PGME, A (? L)
How do we make it happen?	Implementation/change management	CE, A, M, PGME (? L)
Have we got the new treatment working?	Audit of process	A, CE
Is it doing what we wanted it to?	Audit of outcome	A, CE
Is appropriate evidence lacking?	Research questions	R, CE
Is it value for effort?		
Is it value for resources?	Economics and statistics	S, E
Is it the best use of resources?		

CE = clinical epidemiology and public health; M = management; A = audit; R = research; L = library; S = statistician; E = economist.

References

1. SANDERSON, C. (1996) *Evidence-based Candidates for the Audit and Purchasing Agenda [Report].* North Thames Regional Health Authority, London. Cited in Bandolier 1996; 3(3) (Number 25): 5.
2. ROYAL COLLEGE OF PHYSICIANS (1989) *Fractured neck of femur, prevention and management: summary and recommendations of a report of the Royal College of Physicians.* J. Roy. Coll. Phys. 23: 8–12.
3. AUDIT COMMISSION (1995) *United They Stand: Co-ordinating Care for Elderly Patients with Hip Fracture.* HMSO, London.
4. TODD, C.J., FREEMAN, C.J., CAMILLERI-FERRANTE, C. et al. (1995) *Differences in mortality after fracture of the hip: the East Anglian audit.* Br. Med. J. 310: 904–8.
5. BEDFORD, M. (1996) *Broken hips – measuring performance.* Bandolier Number 25, Vol 3 (issue 3): 4
6. FREEMANTLE, N., GRILL, I.R., GRIMSHAW, J.M. and OXMAN, A.D. (1995) *Implementing the findings of medical research: the Cochrane Collaboration and effective professional practice.* Quality in Health Care 4: 45–7.
7. FREEMANTLE, N., HENRY, D., MAYNARD, A. and TORRANCE, G. (1995) *Promoting cost-effective prescribing.* Br. Med. J. 310: 995–6.
8. SUMMERTON, N. (1995) *The burden of proof.* Health Service J. Number 5481 (30.11.95), Vol 105: 33

7.2   EVIDENCE-BASED PRIMARY CARE

Primary care is that form of care to which the patient can gain access directly. It comprises primary medical care, community nursing and those aspects of mental health and learning disability services that are delivered to people at home. For every million population in the UK, there are about 250 general practice or community care sites, compared with only 3–4 hospitals; for every million population, about 20 million clinical decisions will be made each year in primary care.

There are several important differences between primary care and hospital-based care.

- A wider range of health problems is seen.
- The professionals who work within primary care are scattered geographically: a hospital may comprise one or two sites, whereas primary care professionals may work at 100–200.
- Many important decisions have to be made in a patient's home.
- Access to a library is difficult and the support of a librarian is rarely available.

For these reasons, evidence-based decision making is more difficult to organise in primary care; however, the immensity of the task need not lead to paralysis. Although the range of problems encountered is wide, only a small number of problems commonly occur and the organisation of evidence for these common problems is a manageable task. In one study of decision making in general practice in the UK, it was found that the effective treatment of the health problems of a large proportion of patients has already been determined on the basis of evidence. A total of 122 consecutive doctor–patient consultations conducted over 2 days was reviewed; 21 were excluded because of insufficient data while the remaining 101 were assigned to one of three evidence base categories (see Table 7.3).[1]

Table 7.3   (Source: Gill et al[1])

Evidence base	No. consultations
RCTs	31
Convincing non-experimental evidence, e.g. incision and drainage of an abscess	51
Interventions without substantial evidence	19

When making decisions about mental health and learning disability services or about individuals who have these healthcare needs, a small number of common problems recurs and the evidence base can therefore be constrained to a manageable size.

7.2.1   Improving access: promoting finding

Those whose job it is to provide evidence to decision makers must:

- ensure easy access to information;
- provide relevant information, i.e. minimise the amount disseminated to the busy primary care professional.

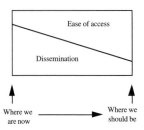

1. Ease of access: it can take hours for a primary care professional to reach and use a library and return to base, but access to that same information can be achieved by phone, fax, Wide Area Network or the Internet, provided the service of a good librarian is available.
2. Relevant information: MEDLINE and EMBASE are excellent resources but they may generate a large volume of detailed information inappropriate to decision making in primary and community care, principally because most of the articles have been written by researchers for researchers. Primary care and community professionals need distillates of primary research related to the clinical problems they encounter, that is, evidence-based guidelines and the facility to access the evidence directly if necessary (see Table 7.4).

Table 7.4 Need for and availability of different types of clinical information

Type of clinical information	Primary care need	Availability
Evidence-based guidelines	++++	+
Written abstract of the systematic review on which the guideline is based	+++	++
Data from the systematic review	++	++
Primary research on which the systematic review is based	+	++++

Access to information can be facilitated by:

- using computer resources intended for management and administration also to provide evidence to decision makers;
- using a Web page, with access by a separate telephone line to protect primary care information systems' confidentiality;
- regularly downloading information for storage on the primary care hard disks to minimise the dependence on slow Internet connections;
- providing every primary and community care site with a copy of The Cochrane Library (Appendix I);
- ensuring on-line access to MEDLINE, for example, via the BMA library;
- disseminating systematically any new information of high quality needed by primary care decision makers, for instance, in a newsletter;
- ensuring that every primary and community care professional has the support of a librarian for the development of searching and storing skills.

7.2.2 Improving appraisal skills

As primary care professionals have to deal with a wide range of problems, they need a broad evidence base and must be taught the skills of appraisal. Although the approach that needs to be taken is no different from that for decision makers in a hospital, they may benefit from different examples.

Bandolier is a newsletter that is written principally to help clinicians, managers and purchasers develop their appraisal skills; one target audience is general practitioners. The objectives of publishing Bandolier are shown in Box 7.6.

Box 7.6

The objectives of the editors of *Bandolier* are to support any decision maker in their ability to:

- find the best available evidence on tests and treatments;
- be conversant with the criteria used to appraise trials and systematic reviews on tests and clinical and cost effectiveness;
- define absolute and relative risk and be aware of the strengths and weaknesses of different methods of expressing research results;
- define, calculate and use NNT;
- list screening tests that do more good than harm;
- define odds ratios and know their value;
- define and interpret confidence intervals and power;
- distinguish sensitivity, specificity and predictive value of tests.

7.2.3 Building a primary care 'library'

As primary care is often delivered in a patient's home, primary care professionals are dependent upon easy access to information. To be of use, information must be stored in convenient systems. Access to information can be promoted by:

- providing evidence-based guidelines, with the evidence itself easily available;
- offering primary care professionals reference management software;
- giving new professionals high-quality evidence relevant to the job they have to do;
- providing information in various media, e.g.:
  - in Filofax size on paper;
  - in a form that can be downloaded to a personal organiser or other palm top;
  - in hypertext files for a PC or Macintosh;
  - as cue card software that can come up on the screen when the primary care system is running patient record software.

Reference

1. GILL, P., DOWELL, A.C., NEAL, R.D., SMITH, N., HEYWOOD, P. and WILSON, A.C. (1996) *Evidence based general practice: a retrospective study of interventions in one training practice.* Br. Med. J. 312: 819–21.

7.3 EVIDENCE-BASED PURCHASING AND COMMISSIONING

In the provision of healthcare, a trend to separate purchasers from providers appears to be a worldwide phenomenon. This approach enables purchasers to focus on how best to use their finite resources with respect to:

- particular groups of patients;
- particular diseases, such as heart disease;
- particular interventions, such as hip replacement.

Purchasers must make decisions about which health services to buy; providers strive to deliver the best value healthcare to individual patients within the resources available.

7.3.1 Evidence-based needs assessment

A useful definition of a need for evidence-based purchasing is: a health problem for which there is an intervention for which there is strong evidence based on good-quality research that it does more good than harm.

Needs assessment has two stages:

1. estimation of the frequency of various health problems in a population;
2. examination of the evidence for the beneficial and harmful effects of those interventions used to treat each health problem – the focus of this book.

Those who purchase healthcare in the UK experience certain advantages and disadvantages in comparison with purchasers elsewhere in the world. One major disadvantage is that in many parts of the UK there is no or only limited choice of providers when compared with, for example, the USA. However, purchasers in the UK have the major advantage of covering discrete populations; in the USA or in some European countries, the population of a single city may be covered by three or more nationwide purchasers. This advantage of being able to focus on a discrete population confers upon UK purchasers the broader role of health 'commissioners' who have the ability to supplement what is achieved by negotiation with providers during the contracting process with:

- the promotion of health generally;
- public and patient education;
- professional education, thereby exerting an influence through the resources invested in education;
- commissioning research where evidence is lacking, thereby exerting an influence through the Research and Development levy.

Purchasers can use their purchasing powers in conjunction with the supplementary levers for change listed above to accomplish four evidence-based tasks:

1. resource reallocation among disease management systems;
2. resource reallocation within a single disease management system;
3. managing innovation;
4. controlling increases in healthcare costs without affecting the health of the population.

7.3.2 Resource reallocation between disease management systems

A disease management system consists of all those services and interventions designed to improve the health of individuals who have a particular disease, such as diabetes, or a group of diseases, such as cardiac disease. Such systems can be managed by the use of guidelines, for both the referral and discharge of patients (see 1–3 in Fig. 7.5), and for the treatment of patients (see A–D in Fig. 7.5). If all the elements of a system are governed by the use of guidelines the care delivered is often referred to as 'managed care'.

In the NHS, disease management systems are rudimentary because the service is still dominated by broad distinctions between primary and secondary care or between hospital and community care. It is impossible to make an evidence-based decision about the balance of expenditure between primary and secondary care as a whole; it is only possible to make evidence-based decisions about the balance of expenditure on primary and secondary care for a particular disease. A comparison of the health

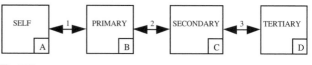

Fig. 7.5

outcomes from investment in different disease management systems requires information from studies of safety, effectiveness and cost, for example, by comparing the cost per QALY.

However, purchasers are not usually asked to reallocate resources on the basis of specific diseases; the purchase of healthcare is usually founded on contracts for particular patient groups, and purchasers face demands to increase the amount of investment in the ENT, the oral surgery or the gynaecology contract (sometimes all three). If purchasers can address only the secondary care sector of these systems, it is worth asking the following questions.

- What would be the beneficial health effects of adding £200 000 to each of these three contracts?
- What would be the health effects of subtracting £200 000 from each of these three contracts?

In both cases, it is wise to elicit the evidence upon which any answers have been based.

7.3.3   Resource reallocation within a single disease management system

Any decision maker trying to reallocate resources within a disease management system on the basis of evidence that resources could be better spent faces several problems.

- Increased expenditure in budget A, such as the drug budget, is required before there can be savings in budget B, the in-patient budget.
- The budgets may be in different compartments (although the introduction of GP fundholding in the UK has brought drug and hospital care budgets together for fundholders).
- The potential savings may appear to be large when calculated nationally; for instance, increasing the prescription of ACE inhibitors in general practice will reduce hospital costs for the treatment of heart failure, but for an individual hospital the actual reduction in the amount of resources used may not be sufficient to allow a facility, such as a ward, to be closed and 'real' cash to be released for reallocation into another part of the system.

These problems are particularly difficult for purchasers to address because:

- they are not able to reduce expenditure on hospital care and redirect it into primary care drug budgets;
- they may not have access to diagnostic service costs, which are not subject to external contract but allocated internally within a provider unit;
- professionals in any service in which savings from better management of one disease have been made can usually identify other needs among a different group of patients in their care which they believe should be met with these resources; for example, professionals in a respiratory unit would argue that any savings on hospital care of asthma should be spent on sleep apnoea or cystic fibrosis.

The main opportunities for better disease management within a hospital are open to the managers at that hospital. However, it is possible for health 'commissioners' to promote disease management systems by focusing on specific points on the primary/secondary care interface, rather than making broad generalisations about need for closer co-operation between the two sectors. Within a single disease management system, a purchaser will attempt to promote cost containment on the basis of research evidence and to minimise any adverse effects on the health of the population (Fig. 7.6).

7.3.4   Managing innovation

Innovation occurs continually. A purchaser must try to manage the introduction of innovation such that:

- those innovations that do more good than harm, and which are affordable, are introduced at a particular standard of quality – *promoting innovation*;
- those innovations that do more harm than good are not introduced – *stopping starting*;
- innovations of unknown effect are investigated during trials – *promoting trials*.

7.3.4.1 Promoting innovation

Promoting innovation has two facets:

1. promoting completely novel interventions;
2. promoting a novel way of delivering an established service.

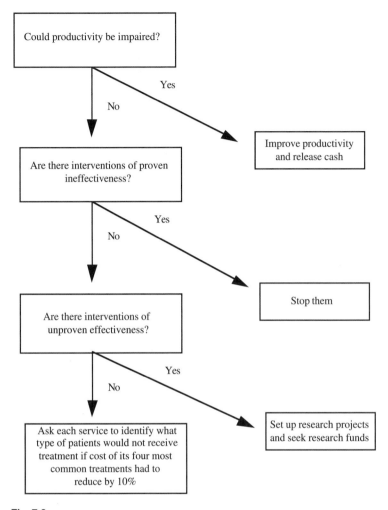

Fig. 7.6
Evidence-based cost containment or cutting

When promoting a novel intervention, for example, thrombolysis after acute myocardial infarction (AMI), it is possible for purchasers to be explicit about their requirements when negotiating contracts. It is more problematic when trying to change established professional practice, for instance, persuading gynaecologists to stop performing dilatation and curettage (D&C) operations in women under the age of 40 years, or to perform fewer Caesarean sections.

Although this can be specified in a contract, other means of promoting change have to be used to reinforce contract specifications, namely:

- professional education and audit;
- public and patient education;
- the development of better systems of care.

The development of better systems of care is particularly important in situations in which a change in professional practice is not sufficient to ensure a better outcome for patients: for example, for thrombolysis after AMI to be delivered effectively, a reconfiguration of the system of care is necessary to change various facets of how patients with chest pain are managed when they contact their GP, when they are in transit in the ambulance and when they arrive at the A&E department.

7.3.4.2 Stopping starting

When there is no evidence (from good-quality research) that an intervention does more good than harm, it should not be introduced. In such situations, it is vital for purchasers to be clear about innovations they do not wish to purchase for a particular population, not because of cost but because of the lack of evidence of effectiveness.

The logic is easy for press and public to understand: all interventions are associated with risk; some people will suffer if any intervention is introduced; if there is no evidence of a beneficial effect, the harm done by the intervention will be greater than the good.

Interventions of proven ineffectiveness and unproven effectiveness should be clearly identified. If any intervention in the latter group is introduced, it must be only as part of a properly designed and ethically approved trial.

7.3.4.3   Promoting trials

Interventions of unproven effectiveness should be tested within an RCT; purchasers should promote and support the performance of RCTs. One benefit of promoting trials is it enables those who pay for healthcare to be categorical about which services/interventions will be supported. For example, in the UK, the NHS Executive (NHSE) issued an Executive Letter (EL) about improving the effectiveness of clinical services [EL(95)105], as part of their strategy for improving clinical effectiveness. In Annex 1 of the EL, the NHSE was explicit about which interventions were included in the Health Technology Assessment Programme and gave clear advice as follows.

'The following interventions are currently under assessment (or studies will start in the next 12 months). Purchasers are advised to invest in these interventions in the context of the assessment but not as part of routine care. It is important that sufficient numbers of patients are recruited to these clinical studies to reduce areas of uncertainty. Purchasers should therefore play an active role and encourage providers to participate fully in recognised assessments.

The following assessments include major clinical trials and systematic reviews. These studies are supported by the Medical Research Council, the Department of Health, charities and the NHS (including the NHS Health Technology Assessment Programme). These have been grouped together in broad service categories, for convenience.

Briefing sheets for each of the interventions listed are available from the contact given at the end of this annex. This should place the assessment in context and better inform purchasing practice.'

Included in Annex 1 were those screening tests that should not be offered as part of 'routine care' but should be supported 'in the context of the assessment', i.e. offered only as part of a high-quality research programme (see Box 7.7).

Box 7.7 Screening tests which should be offered only within the context of research (UK)

- Screening for colorectal cancer by once only flexible sigmoidoscopy
- Antenatal screening for HIV
- Screening for Down's syndrome, using ultrasound measurement of nuchal translucency
- Screening for fragile X
- Neonatal screening for inborn errors of metabolism, including use of tandem mass-spectrometry and DNA analysis
- Screening for abdominal aortic aneurysm
- Screening for ovarian cancer
- Breast cancer screening from the age of 40
- Yearly breast screening
- Identifying and monitoring osteoporosis, featuring use of:
  - dual-energy X-ray absorptiometry;
  - low frequency ultrasound;
  - biochemical markers.

Box 7.8 GRiPP Topics

- The use of corticosteroids for women in preterm labour
- The management of services to prevent and treat stroke
- The use of D&C for dysfunctional uterine bleeding in women under 40 years of age
- The use of grommets for children with glue ear
- Thrombolysis for people with acute myocardial infarction

7.3.5 GRiPP – getting research into purchasing and practice

The GRiPP project was originated within the Oxford Regional Health Authority in 1993.[1] Initially, five specific therapeutic interventions were selected for which there was good research evidence of effectiveness and appropriateness, but about which there was a gap between what was known and what was practised in the service (see Box 7.8). Each therapeutic intervention was adopted by one of the four district health authorities in the region. The lessons learned from the GRiPP project are shown in Appendix V.

Although a lot of effort went into achieving small changes in these five areas, one of the most important outcomes was the impact that the GRiPP project had on the culture of the organisation. By focusing on specific treatments for which there was a strong research evidence base, the concept of evidence-based decision making and the need to use evidence in all decisions was adopted much more quickly than would have been the case if general exhortations to practise evidence-based decision making had been made.

7.3.6 Evidence-based insurance

In the past, the source of finance has dictated the system of healthcare introduced. In countries in which systems of paying for healthcare develop, there are two main sources of finance:

1. insurance;
2. taxation.

In some countries, there may be complicated permutations of these two systems, for example, government underwriting of insurance schemes. Insurance-based systems derive revenue from customers; in tax-based systems, health services are paid for directly from funds raised through taxation. The distinction between the two systems has changed dramatically in recent years. Some insurance companies provide their own healthcare, for example, in health maintenance organisations such as Kaiser Permanente. In tax-based systems, such as the NHS, the opposite trend is taking place, as demonstrated by the division between the purchase and provision of healthcare.

Insurance schemes operate in a different way from health authorities in the NHS. Instead of negotiating contracts for services for geographical populations, there are health plans which cover those people (sometimes called the 'members') who pay the premiums of the insurance company.

In the past, insurance companies paid all the costs of treatment, but as costs have increased the services provided have been rationed; the plans insurance companies now offer are carefully couched in what Eddy calls 'benefit language', namely, that part of the contract between a plan and its members that describes the interventions or benefits for which the plan will pay. 'Benefit language' in which health plans are expressed has three main components:[2]

1. coverage categories describing the services that will be covered – for example, orthopaedic surgery is covered but not osteopathy;
2. patient responsibilities – the contribution the member may have to make to the cost of care;
3. coverage criteria.

Coverage criteria are the means by which the insurance companies fine-tune the categories of service covered and seek to balance cost control and the provision of a range of services that members will find attractive. It is upon these coverage criteria that guidelines, protocols and clinical policies are developed by insurance companies, and thus it is through coverage criteria that a system of 'managed care' is created (see Section 7.3.2).

The coverage criteria will vary from one health plan to another. They relate not to services but to specific therapeutic interventions, namely, activities that prevent, diagnose, treat or improve a medical condition. The criteria that must be met for an intervention to be included in a health plan are shown in Box 7.9.

Coverage criteria are the means insurers use to promote evidence-based healthcare, in particular, through the requirement that 'sufficient evidence' is available. Sufficient evidence was the concept investigated in the studies of the proportion of patients whose care is determined by evidence shown in Table 7.3 and Table 9.1. Sufficient evidence is defined as that evidence derived from RCTs and systematic reviews of trials and convincing non-experimental evidence (e.g. there is convincing empirical evidence to support the decision to drain an abscess) (see Table 4.2).

Clinicians in the UK have worked within a form of managed care since 1948. The development of a system of managed care has occurred rapidly in the USA. In less than two decades, American doctors have been taken from a tradition in which they worked as they chose to a system of care that is governed by stricter controls than are set out in UK purchasing contracts. In one editorial published in the *Annals of Internal Medicine*, the situation was described as

---

Box 7.9 Coverage criteria (Source: Eddy[2])

- The intervention is used for a medical condition
- There is sufficient evidence to draw conclusions about the intervention's effects on health outcomes
- The evidence demonstrates that the intervention can be expected to produce its intended effects on health outcomes
- The intervention's expected beneficial effects on health outcomes outweigh its expected harmful effects
- The intervention is the most cost-effective method available to address the medical condition

follows: 'the physician has moved from Pegasus, soaring aloft on the heady excitement of biomedical science, to Sisyphus, condemned forever to push a boulder up a hill'.[3]

7.3.7   'Black belt' decision making

The approach described hitherto is relatively simple but complicated flow charts can be used; an example of one is shown in Fig. 7.7.

References

1. DUNNING, M., McQUAY, H. and MILNE, R. (1994) *Getting a GRiP*. Health Service J., Number 5400 (28.4.94), Vol. 104: 24–6.
2. EDDY, D. (1996) *Benefit language. Criteria that will improve quality while reducing cost*. JAMA 275: 650–7.
3. LIPKIN, M. Jr. (1996) *Sisyphus or Pegasus? The physician interviewer in the era of corporatization of care*. Ann. Intern. Med. 124: 511–12.

7.4 PROMOTING CLINICAL EFFECTIVENESS IN THE NHS

In the UK, the Department of Health set up an R&D programme in 1991 which had five main functions:

1. to ascertain the knowledge that NHS decision makers need;
2. to ensure that knowledge was produced;
3. to make the knowledge available to decision makers;
4. to promote the implementation of R&D findings;
5. to promote an evaluative culture.

The key verb is ' to promote' in functions 4 and 5. Within the R&D Programme, the aim is primarily that of producing knowledge which is needed and making that knowledge available. To complement this activity, the Secretary of State for Health launched a Clinical Effectiveness Initiative which has a simple and easily understood framework with three main themes:

1. inform;
2. change;
3. monitor.

As the primary purpose of the NHS is 'to secure through the resources available, the greatest possible improvement to the health of the people', it was emphasised that providing

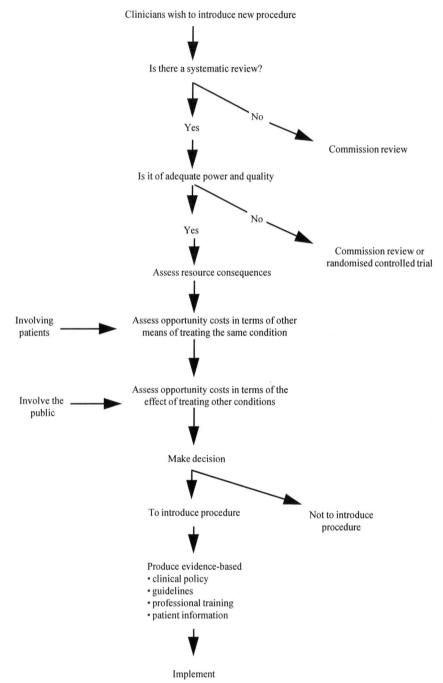

Fig. 7.7
Flow chart of decision making based on research synthesis (Source: Chalmers and Irwig[4], see p 181)

services that are effective in terms of result and cost was central to achieving this purpose.

The Clinical Effectiveness Initiative brings together several separate projects and programmes. In the booklet produced for chief executives, the ways in which a wide range of Departmental initiatives within the service could be brought together to increase the cost-effectiveness of the NHS are described. This bold programme of work has been built upon the R&D initiative to ensure that research-based knowledge is not only produced and made available to decision makers but also used as evidence in decision making to improve the health service and the health of the population.

7.5 EVIDENCE-BASED POLICY MAKING

Policy: '5. a course of action adopted and pursued by a government, party, ruler, statesman, etc.; any course of action adopted as advantageous or expedient. (The chief living sense.)'

Shorter Oxford English Dictionary

'There is nothing a politician likes so little as to be well informed; it makes decision making so complex and difficult.'

J. M. Keynes

Policies relating to the delivery of healthcare can be categorised into two types:

1. policies on the financing and organisation of healthcare;
2. public health policies.

For policies on financing and organisation of healthcare, there is little available evidence; for public health policies, more evidence is available and there is a greater tradition of using evidence in decision making.

Politics tends to be driven by beliefs, and it is the values politicians believe to be important that dominate decision making. Such decisions will be tempered by the availability of resources, the allocation of which may also be based on beliefs. Evidence also plays a part in policy making, but some policies have been made without consideration of the evidence available.*

* However, in the UK, during the 1990s, there was a significant shift in political interest to endorsing the principles of evidence-based decision making. This was manifest by support for the National Research and Development Programme in which there was commitment not only to producing new knowledge but also to basing healthcare decisions on knowledge. In 1995, the Government promoted the practice of evidence-based medicine in the delivery of healthcare within the NHS, and, in 1996, the principle that high-quality knowledge should be central to healthcare provision was identified as one of three strategic themes that would be used to guide the NHS into the next century.

7.5.1 Budgetary pressures – the begetter of evidence

Times, indeed, are changing, principally as a result of budgetary pressures, as illustrated by this eloquent letter written by Danial Patrick Moynihan, Chairman of the US Senate Finance Committee.[1]

'Dear Dr Tyson,

You will recall that last Thursday when you so kindly joined us at a meeting of the Democratic Policy Committee you and I discussed the President's family preservation proposal. You indicated how much he supports the measure. I assured you I, too, support it, but went on to ask what evidence was there that it would have any effect. You assured me there was such data. Just for fun, I asked for two citations.

The next day we received a fax from Sharon Glied of your staff with a number of citations and a paper, 'Evaluating the Results', that appears to have been written by Frank Farrow of the Center for the Study of Social Policy here in Washington and Harold Richman at the Chapin Hall Center at the University of Chicago. The paper is quite direct: '...solid proof that family preservation services can affect a state's overall placement rates is still lacking.'

Just yesterday, the same Chapin Hall Center released an 'Evaluation of the Illinois Family First Placement Prevention Program: Final Report'. This was a large-scale study of the Illinois Family First initiative authorized by the Illinois Family Preservation Act of 1987. It was 'designed to test effects of this program on out-of-home placements of children and other outcomes, such as subsequent child maltreatment'. Data on case and service characteristics were provided by Family First caseworkers on approximately 4, 500 cases; approximately 1, 600 families participated in the randomized experiment. The findings are clear enough. 'Overall, the Family First placement prevention program results in a slight increase in placement rates (when data from all experimental sites are combined). This effect disappears once case and site variations are taken into account.' In other words, there are either negative effects or no effects.'

In this case, the shortage of resources forced policy makers to collect evidence and change policy.

7.5.2   Policies on health service financing and organisation

At the highest level, any government can decide on the level of investment in health services that will be made by that government. However, policy makers also make decisions about the organisation of health services, which are usually related to the financing of health services. In the NHS, examples of organisational policy making include:

- the creation of health authorities in 1974, in which were combined the financing of the local authority health committee and the regional hospital boards;
- the introduction of the purchaser/provider split and the creation of GP fundholding in 1991;
- the abolition of regional health authorities in 1996.

In these organisational changes, many of which have taken place since the inception of the NHS in 1948, power changed hands, an outcome achieved principally by changing the responsibility for resources.

Each organisational change may be instigated to fulfil one or more objectives, such as:

- to decentralise power;
- to involve more people in decision making;
- to encourage cost control;
- to reduce the number of managerial staff;
- to encourage competition as a stimulus to reduce costs and increase quality.

Although such objectives and the type of organisational change introduced may reflect the ideology of the political party in power, they can be based on evidence. The evidence may sometimes be the experience of what happened since the last change in funding and organisation; sometimes it is

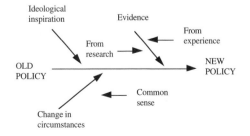

based on research findings. The idea for a new policy may also be generated by an individual, a pressure group or a think tank; it will probably also reflect their political ideology. Often, policy initiatives can also be supported by common sense: sometimes, it is obvious that a former policy needs to be amended to meet new circumstances.

GP fundholding, for example, was introduced as part of a series of changes designed:

- to increase competitive pressures on the providers of healthcare as a stimulus to improve efficiency and quality;
- to increase the motivation of general practitioners to control expenditure on prescribing by allowing them to retain any 'savings' for other types of patient care.

There was no evidence on which to base such a policy, although it would have been possible to design and manage an RCT of GP fundholding, randomly allocating volunteer practices to be either fundholding or control practices. It was not practicable to perform such a trial because it would have taken 3 or more years to complete and policy makers operate on a timescale that does not generally admit of such delays. Although it would have been feasible to identify pilot practices, as a 'simpler' trial design than an RCT, this strategy would also be unacceptable to policy makers because it could be interpreted as uncertainty about the policy of GP fundholding – uncertainty is not a characteristic policy makers like to display.

The policy of GP fundholding has now been evaluated in several observational cohort studies, in which it was concluded that:

'No evidence existed that budgetary pressures caused first wave fundholders to reduce referral rates, although the method of budget allocation may have encouraged general practitioners to inflate their referral rates in the preparatory year. Despite investment in new practice facilities, no evidence yet exists that fundholding encourages a shift away from specialist care';[2]

'Fundholding has altered practice prescribing patterns compared with those of non-fundholders, increasing generic prescribing and reducing the rate of increase of prescribing costs'.[3]

Despite the usefulness of these studies, they are evaluations of a policy already in place; as such they are examples of policy-based research, not research-based policy. Similarly, a search for research evidence on purchasing healthcare in the UK[4, 5] or on self-governing Trusts[6, 7] will identify only articles on work done after the introduction of such policies.

7.5.2.1   Searching

To find articles on health policy, use the MeSH term 'health policy'.

7.5.2.2   Appraisal

When appraising research evidence on a policy, there are two important questions to ask.

1. How valid is the evaluation?
2. How relevant is the policy to the 'local' service?

A checklist of questions for the appraisal of research designed to evaluate a healthcare policy is shown in Box 7.10.

7.5.2.3   Applicability and relevance

If the evaluation of a policy was carried out in a different country, the issue of relevance is also important.

Box 7.10   Checklist for the appraisal of research designed to evaluate healthcare policy

- Were the explicit policy objectives clearly stated?
- Did the research workers identify and articulate any implicit objectives of the policy under investigation?
- Were valid outcome measures identified for each of the explicit and implicit objectives?
- Was data collection complete?
- Were data collected before and after the introduction of the new policy?
- Was the follow-up of sufficient length to allow the effects of policy change to become evident?
- Were any other factors that could have produced the changes (other than the policy) identified in the key criteria and discussed?
- Were possible sources of bias in the research workers acknowledged by the authors or in accompanying editorials?

There are two aspects to relevance in this situation:

1. the feasibility of introducing a particular policy into one's own country;
2. the practicability of introducing the interventions associated with the implementation of that policy into one's own country.

For example, legislation passed in the USA is of limited relevance to the UK, and vice versa, but the potential effects of legislation on professional behaviour or managerial decision making are relevant and it may be possible to reproduce those in other countries, albeit through different legislation and by other means.

7.5.3 Public health policies

Public health has been defined as the improvement of health through the organised efforts of society – social interventions. The interventions that cannot be undertaken by individual members of the public or individual clinicians include:

- screening programmes;
- immunisation;
- environmental protection.

Screening and immunisation programmes are simple interventions analogous to interventions in clinical practice and should be evaluated by RCTs and systematic reviews of trials (see Sections 5.3 and 5.2, respectively). Environmental protection policies, on the other hand, are a different type of social intervention designed to remove or reduce risk. This requires a two-stage process:

1. establishing that a particular factor, or set of factors, increases the risk of a disease;
2. establishing that policies to reduce risk are feasible, effective and affordable.

7.5.3.1 Does the evidence show an increased risk?

Risk factor analysis is commonly required in public health to determine whether a cluster of cases of a particular condition has occurred by chance or constitutes an 'epidemic' that has an environmental cause. In epidemiological research, risk factors can be identified and quantified within cohort studies (Section 5.5) and case-control studies (Section 5.4); however, personnel in service public health departments are often asked about a health hazard which may have been publicised by the media – for example, a public perception that there has been a rapid increase in the incidence of childhood leukaemia related to, or reported in the media as 'caused by', electricity power lines.

It is relatively easy to answer such queries if evidence is available from cohort or case-control studies or an expert is on hand who can give a scientific briefing based on the strength of evidence about the magnitude of the risk. It is more difficult when a director of public health is faced with the media eager to know if there is an epidemic of a particular cancer, what the cause is and what the health service is doing about it. The incidence of every non-communicable disease fluctuates with time; when the disease is uncommon and numbers of sufferers are small, fluctuations that would be unremarkable if large numbers of cases occurred regularly can appear to be dramatic. In this situation, a director of public health must decide whether the increase in incidence is greater than that which would be expected by chance.

Statistical techniques for the analysis of disease clusters can be exceptionally difficult to perform; indeed, the use of some techniques is limited to those who have degrees in mathematics and statistics. It is, however, essential for public health policy makers to understand the application of various techniques in the analysis of clusters of disease – sometimes called 'extreme data'. The most accessible and comprehensible paper on the subject is by Palmer.[8] He describes a simple method that can be used to measure the 'degree of surprise' to patterns of data classified by time and place. This method will help any decision maker presented with such data detect 'significant departures from random variation'.[8]

Palmer based this paper on a real health problem. In one health region of the UK (when there was a configuration of 14 regional health authorities), one of the eight health districts in that region had the highest annual incidence of a particular disease on four occasions in 6 years. There was an obvious need to identify whether this was a cause for concern (a 'surprise') or simply due to chance. The approach Palmer took to determine this point will become increasingly important as league tables of performance are published: he reviewed conventional techniques used to analyse disease clusters, such as longitudinal data analysis and the Friedman two-way analysis of variance, and presented a simple easily understandable alternative.

He warns against placing too much emphasis on the probability level of 0.05 – the 'surprise threshold' – because a probability below 0.05 is not impossible, it is simply less likely. Anyone responsible for the health of a population presented with either population-based data on mortality or data relating to the performance of different health services serving that population should either be able to carry out the type of analysis outlined in Palmer's paper or have access to personnel who can do so.

He also identified a trap into which most people fall: focusing solely on the performer at the 'wrong' end of any league table, depending upon whether appearance at the top or bottom indicates a problem. Palmer gives guidance on other statistical approaches that can be used, including the facility to take account of ranking over a period of time, such as the repeated appearance of a provider unit in the worst five of the league table.

7.5.3.2 Is it possible to reduce the risk?

To establish whether a policy designed to reduce risk is feasible, effective and affordable, such as a screening or an immunisation policy, the techniques used to evaluate the effectiveness of a new intervention, that is, those based on a systematic review of the results of RCTs, will provide the best evidence. Difficult as they may be to organise, RCTs of public health interventions should be subjected to the same rigorous appraisal as is applied to clinical interventions. It could be argued that there is a need for stronger evidence because public health interventions are by definition offered to healthy populations; some of the people who receive the intervention will be put at risk from that intervention (because no intervention is without risk), a proportion of whom would not have developed the disease even if the public health programme had not been introduced.

Once a risk to the public health has been identified, a policy maker must decide:

- if an intervention can reduce that risk;
- if it is possible to introduce the intervention(s) necessary to reduce that risk;
- whether the measures taken to reduce the particular risk that is the main cause of concern will increase other risks;
- what the cost would be to save a life or provide an added year of life; cost-effectiveness and cost–utility studies are of particular importance in public health policy making because the costs of prevention can be surprisingly high.

7.5.3.3   The use of legislation to promote public health

The traditional role of law is to protect the individual from harm by third parties.

There is an inverse relationship between the magnitude of a health problem and the strength of opposition to legislation. The relationship between these two variables is shown in Fig. 7.8. When public concern about a problem exceeds public opposition to legislation, the threshold is crossed and policy is made.

However, the level of that threshold can be influenced by many factors other than the magnitude of the health problem, some of which raise the threshold while others lower it. Strength of evidence is now a necessary prerequisite before public health policy can be made, but the converse is not true: public health policy is not necessarily made despite the existence of strong evidence for it.

Greater obstacles are faced when developing a public health policy that seeks to protect individuals from their own inclinations – the paternalistic role of law. Powerful evidence is needed to show that such legislation is not only effective but also safe. When legislation was being drafted to make the wearing of seat belts compulsory, a law that now seems uncontroversial, the argument was made that the state should not introduce paternalistic legislation for the benefit of a large number of people if it resulted in the unnecessary harm of even one person: it was considered tantamount to sacrificing one person for the benefit of other people who did not wish to take protective action of their own volition.

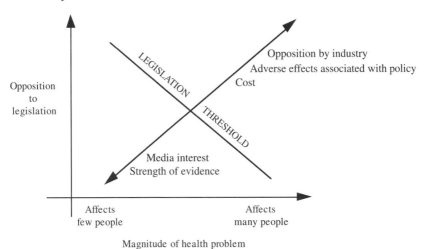

Fig. 7.8
Factors affecting the 'legislation threshold': factors at the right-hand end of the double-headed arrow will raise the threshold whereas those on the left-hand will lower it

There is evidence that controls on cigarette advertising can play a part in preventing teenage smoking, but that evidence is not regarded as strong enough to justify a policy of statutory, as opposed to voluntary, control of advertising. As so often occurs in policy making, values outweigh evidence.

References

1. MOYNIHAN, D.P. (1995) The Congressional Record, 12 December 1995 Reproduced as *Congress builds a coffin*, New York Review of Books, January 11 1996, pp. 33–6.
2. SURENDER, R., BRADLOW, J., COULTER, A., DOLL, H. and STEWART-BROWN, S. (1995). *Prospective study of trends in referral patterns in fundholding and non-fundholding practices in the Oxford Region 1990–1994.* Br. Med. J. 311: 1205–8.
3. WILSON, R.P.H., BUCHAN, I. and WALLEY, T. (1995) *Alterations in prescribing by general practitioners: an observational study.* Br. Med. J. 311: 1347–50.
4. GHODSE, B. (1995) *Extracontractual referrals: safety valve or administrative paperchase?* Br. Med. J. 310: 1573–6.
5. KLEIN, R. and REDMAYNE, S. (1992) *Patterns of Priorities: A Study of the Purchasing and Rationing Policies of Health Authorities.* National Association of Health Authorities and Trusts, Birmingham.
6. SHIELL, A. (1991) *Competing hospitals: assessing the impact of self-governing status in the United Kingdom.* Health Policy 19(2–3): 141–58.
7. SPURGEON, P. (1994) *Purchaser/provider relationships: current practice and future prospects.* Health Service Manage. Res. 7: 195–200.
8. PALMER, C.R. (1993) *Probability of recurrence of extreme data: an aid to decision making.* Lancet 342: 845–7.

7.6 EVIDENCE-BASED LITIGATION

Although the word 'evidence' is much used in court, the evidence that is presented and appraised there and upon which judgements are made is of a different quality to the evidence discussed in this book.

Within the legal system in the UK, great store is laid by expert opinion which is regarded as synonymous with research-based evidence; both the prosecution and the defence try to find the best expert they can, that is, the best expert to support their case, Furthermore, after an expert has given an opinion, its generalisability and relevance to the individual case under judgement appears to be treated with remarkable naivety. Probabilistic thinking is inimical to a system in which the outcome is either 'guilty' or 'not guilty', and its potential contribution in this situation has been emphatically ruled out by the Bench of the Court of Appeal, as the President of the Royal Statistical Society described in his Presidential address.[1]

'Evidence of the Bayes Theorem or any similar statistical method of analysis in a criminal trial plunged the jury into inappropriate and unnecessary realms of theory and complexity, deflecting them from their proper task. ... Their Lordships ... had very grave doubts as to whether that evidence was properly admissible because it trespassed on an area peculiarly and exclusively within the jury's province, namely the way in which they evaluated the relationship between one piece of evidence and another. The Bayes Theorem might be an appropriate and useful tool for statisticians, but it was not appropriate for us in jury trials or as a means to assist the jury in its task.'

In the USA, the situation appears to be worse, as described by Marcia Angell in *Science on Trial*,[2] a brilliant book about the legal management of the purported harmful effects of breast implants. Despite the lack of research-based evidence that breast implants increase the risk of auto-immune disease, a class action amounting to $4.25 billion has evolved. As a result of media and legal hyperbole, supported by 'experts' who have published nothing of note on this subject, more than 400 000 women believe they may have been harmed. Apart from the fact that many lawyers have become fabulously rich working on such cases, the most dispiriting aspect of the saga is the lack of impact the type of evidence that readers of this book might accept actually had on the judges or the jurors. Even that acme of medical science, the *New England Journal of Medicine*, of which Dr Angell is the Executive Editor, was subpoenaed and accused of conspiracy by lawyers when it published the Food and Drug Administration's statement on breast implants[3] and Dr Angell's editorial.[4] In Angell's analysis of attitudes towards science in the USA, she argues that the situation shows no sign of improving as people turn away from science to magic in a world that is becoming increasingly uncertain.

References

1. SMITH, A. (1996) *Mad cows and ecstasy: chance and choice in an evidence-based society.* J.R. Stat. Assoc. A159: 367–83.
2. ANGELL, M. (1996) *Science on trial.* W.W. Norton & Co. Inc., New York.
3. KESSLER, D. (1992) *The basis for the FDA's decision on breast implants.* New. Eng. J. Med. 326: 1713–15.
4. ANGELL, M. (1992) *Breast implants: protection or paternalism?* New. Eng. J. Med. 326: 1695–6.

PROLOGUE 8

Dear Reader,

Empathise with Dr John Hall, son-in-law of William Shakespeare. He wrote an early treatise on effectiveness called 'Select Observations on English Bodies of Eminent Persons in Desperate Diseases', but his observational epidemiology was weak; most of his observations are of single cases. His objectives, however, were good; in the preface to the treatise he reflects, 'we must study all ways possible to find out and appoint medicines of cheap rate and effectual for money is scarce and country people poor…'.

CHAPTER 8

DEVELOPING THE EVIDENCE MANAGEMENT SKILLS OF INDIVIDUALS

> 'No system can make a bad man good but bad systems can frustrate the efforts of good men.'
>
> Gandhi

Although the health service has undergone numerous system changes, it is wise to remember that management, although supported by systems, is a human activity and it is the competence of the individuals within any system that is of major importance. Nonetheless, a high level of competence does not of itself guarantee good performance; performance is also directly related to an individual's motivation and inversely related to the barriers that individual has to overcome.

$$P = \frac{C \times M}{B}$$

where: P = performance
C = competence
M = motivation
B = barriers

In this chapter, the knowledge and skills that individuals require to increase their competence as decision makers are outlined.

8.1 SEARCHING

Issues about which decisions have to be made usually arise without warning or at inconvenient times. In an ideal world, a manager requests a search for evidence from a librarian; in reality, managers often have to find evidence for themselves.

8.1.1 Competencies

Everyone who makes decisions about groups of patients or populations should be able to:

- define and identify the sources of evidence it is appropriate to search for when faced with a particular decision;
- carry out a search of MEDLINE or EMBASE without the help of a librarian and find at least 60% of the reviews or research studies that would be found by a librarian;
- construct simple search strategies on MEDLINE, using Boolean operators ('and' and 'or') for:
  (a) the following healthcare terms:
    - treatment;
    - test;
    - screening programme;
  (b) the following service characteristics:
    - effectiveness;
    - safety;
    - acceptability;
    - appropriateness;
    - quality;
    - cost-effectiveness;
- download the end-products of a search onto reference management software (Section 8.3).

8.1.2 Training

All decision makers should receive induction training on how to find research evidence. Initial training, however, is effective only if it is supplemented by refresher sessions. For instance, it is advisable for every decision maker to do a search and review it with a skilled searcher several times a year.

8.1.3 Scanning

Evidence can also be found by scanning, that is, regularly reading certain journals. As this can be time consuming, it is wise to decide how much time to spend reading each week and then develop an appropriate scanning strategy (see Box 4.1, p 65).

8.2 APPRAISING EVIDENCE

In future, librarians will be trained to appraise evidence as well as to search for it, and to teach both skills. At present, the main source of appraisal skills is in departments of public health. As a consultant in public health may not always be available when an appraisal needs to be undertaken, all those who make decisions about populations or groups of patients need to have the skills to appraise research articles on healthcare, that is, take a scientific approach to healthcare management.

8.2.1 Competencies

Every decision maker needs to be able to appraise the evidence presented in a review article on the following interventions:

- a therapy (see Section 3.1);
- a test (see Section 3.2);
- a screening programme (see Section 3.3);
- health policy or management changes (see Section 3.4).

Decision makers also need to be able to appraise the quality of the following research methodologies:

- systematic reviews (see Section 5.2);
- RCTs (see Section 5.3);
- qualitative research (see Section 5.8);
- case-control studies (see Section 5.4);
- surveys (see Section 5.6) or cohort studies (see Section 5.5).

Decision makers must also be able to assess the performance or outcomes of an intervention against the following criteria:

- acceptability;
- effectiveness (see Section 6.3);
- safety (see Section 6.4);
- patient satisfaction (see Section 6.5);
- cost-effectiveness (see Section 6.6);
- quality (see Section 6.7);
- appropriateness (see Section 6.8).

These appraisals must also be conducted within the context of 'local' circumstances; a decision maker must consider not only the applicability of the findings to a particular population but also 'local' factors that may affect the outcomes of applying those findings.

For those who do not appraise research evidence regularly, the checklists provided at the book's Web site may be used as prompts whenever appraisal is undertaken. http://www.ihs.ox.ac.uk/ebh.html

8.2.2 Training

The skills of appraisal should be developed during the basic training of all professionals. At present, these skills are virtually ignored; very few decision makers have been taught how to be systematic in their appraisal of a report or a research project. For example, only two of the Royal Colleges, General Practitioners and Psychiatrists, include critical appraisal in their final examinations.

All healthcare organisations need a critical appraisal skills programme (see Appendix IIIB).

8.3 STORING AND RETRIEVING

> 'My storage system? I've got a foot and a half of papers torn out of the BMJ in a pile on my dining-room table.'
>
> A physician, 2 years after graduation

Storing paper is easy, at least in the short term. However, the young doctor quoted above could face problems in 20 years' time if his rate of acquisition continues at 9 inches (22.86 cm) per year. He could probably cope with three four-drawer filing cabinets, storing papers alphabetically by surname of the first author, for example. The drawback with such a filing system, however, is that retrieval is difficult unless the storer has a good memory or the author of the paper has a memorable name. Retrieval from an alphabetically or chronologically based filing system is more difficult if the task is to retrieve all the papers on a particular subject. Although papers or reference cards can be stored by disease grouping, concepts or patient groups, it is not possible to combine any of these categories using a paper-based storage system, e.g. to retrieve all the papers describing trials of coronary heart disease prevention on one occasion and then to retrieve all the papers investigating coronary heart disease in women on another. Only computer-based storage systems have the potential to store useful information in a form that will allow retrieval from several different 'entry' points.

8.3.1 Competencies

Every decision maker should be able to:

- enter references and abstracts, using self-selected keywords, into one of the electronic systems for reference management (Appendix IV);
- search for references within a reference management system;

- download sets of references from the reference management software onto paper.

There are several different types of reference management software available. As professionals within a health service are highly 'mobile', it is vital that every librarian is able to support staff using any of the common reference management software irrespective of the system used in the library.

8.3.2 Training

After a short period of induction training, anyone who is intelligent enough to be a decision maker in a health service should be able to use reference management systems.

8.4 THE 'COMPLEAT' HEALTHCARE MANAGER

> 'The philosophers have only interpreted the world in various ways; the point is to change it.'
>
> Karl Marx

Although searching, appraising and storing (SAS) skills are necessary, they are not sufficient; decision makers also need to practise and improve their skills of implementing research findings if they are to change the organisation of a health service and the patterns of delivery of clinical care.

Although the focus of this book is primarily on developing SAS skills, the skills of implementing the changes that evidence dictates are of equal importance. Many of these are general management skills, such as are necessary for project management or effective team work. Most managers already have these skills because they are developed during management training. As the 21st century approaches, it is the combination of these two sets of skills that will fit any healthcare manager for the challenges ahead.

> General management skills
> +
> Skills for evidence-based decision making
> =
> The 'compleat' healthcare manager

PROLOGUE 9

Dear Reader,

Empathise with Stephen Jay Gould.

'In July 1982, I learned that I was suffering from abdominal mesothelioma, a rare and serious cancer usually associated with exposure to asbestos. When I revived after surgery, I asked my first question of my doctor and chemotherapist: 'What is the best technical literature about mesothelioma?'. She replied, with a touch of diplomacy (the only departure she has ever made from direct frankness), that the medical literature contained nothing really worth reading.

Of course, trying to keep an intellectual away from literature works about as well as recommending chastity to Homo sapiens, *the sexiest primate of all. As soon as I could walk, I made a beeline for Harvard's Countway medical library and punched mesothelioma into the computer's bibliographic search program. An hour later, surrounded by the latest literature on abdominal mesothelioma, I realised with a gulp why my doctor had offered that humane advice. The literature couldn't have been more brutally clear: mesothelioma is incurable, with a median mortality of only 8 months after discovery. I sat stunned for about 15 minutes, then smiled and said to myself: so that's why they didn't give me anything to read.*

Then my mind started to work again, thank goodness…

The problem may be briefly stated: what does 'median mortality of 8 months' signify in our vernacular? I suspect that most people, without training in statistics, would read such a statement as 'I will probably be dead in 8 months' – the very conclusion that must be avoided, both because this formulation is false and because attitude matters so much.'

Stephen Jay Gould,
'The median isn't the message'
in Adam's Navel, 1995

Commentary

Stephen Jay Gould, world-class geologist, baseball guru and beautiful writer, is not perhaps the average patient, but neither should his experience, attitude and skills be disregarded. The patients of the future will be more literate, better organised and better educated than those of today, and many of them will be better at finding, but not necessarily appraising, knowledge using the World Wide Web. The relationship between clinician and patient will continue to evolve and clinicians should be prepared to encounter more patients like Stephen Jay Gould in future.

CHAPTER 9

EVIDENCE-BASED PATIENT CHOICE AND CLINICAL PRACTICE

Every year, for every million population receiving health services, many decisions are made, including:

- hundreds of purchasing decisions;
- thousands of managerial decisions;
- millions of clinical decisions.

9.1 CLINICAL DECISIONS AS DRIVERS OF HEALTHCARE

Clinical decisions are the product of healthcare. They are of direct and immediate importance to patients, but they are also of importance to those who manage and fund health services: one outcome of clinical decision making is expenditure by health services. It has been shown that in a system in which resources are not finite changes in the volume and intensity of clinical practice constitute the major factor driving the increase in healthcare costs that can be controlled.[1]

Although other factors, such as population ageing and the general rate of inflation (Fig. 2.5), increase the cost of healthcare, it is not possible for health service managers to contain these costs. Medical price inflation, another factor increasing costs, can be controlled, by evidence-based purchasing of drugs and equipment, for instance. However, changes in the volume and intensity of clinical practice are factors over which managers can exert considerable influence (see Sections 2.2 and 2.3).

In order to exercise this influence, it is essential for those who make decisions about groups of patients or populations to understand how clinicians, in consultation with their patients, make and take decisions.

Reference

1. EDDY, D.M. (1993) *Three battles to watch in the 1990s*. JAMA 270: 520–6.

9.2 TYPES OF CLINICAL DECISION

9.2.1 'Faceless' decision making

'Faceless' decisions are those in which the decision is based on either a specimen taken from, or an image taken of, a patient. Such decisions are the clinician's interpretation of a test result, sample or image; there is no discussion with the patient or their relatives. As the clinician is a human and not a mechanical instrument, the decision will be influenced not only by what can be seen or measured but also by other factors (see Fig. 9.1, left-hand side).

Owing to the influence of these other factors, 'faceless' decisions are always characterised by:

- interobserver variability: different clinicians decide upon a different interpretation of the same image or test results;
- intraobserver variability: the same clinician decides upon a different interpretation of the same image or test results on different occasions.

These characteristics of 'faceless' decision making can be observed among even the best clinicians; moreover, variability increases as the image or test result approaches 'borderline'. Although certain levels of inter- and intraobserver variability are unacceptable and must be eradicated through clinical audit, inter- and intraobserver variability are inevitable consequences of using human beings as measuring and decision-taking instruments (Section 3.2.1).

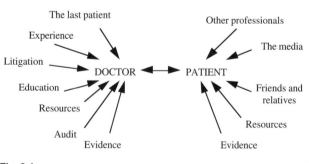

Fig. 9.1
The decision drivers

9.2.2 Face-to-face decision making

The principal characteristic distinguishing face-to-face decisions is the dialogue between clinician and patient, to which the patient will bring their own set of beliefs, attitudes and values. Consequently, there are many more variables involved when face-to-face decisions are made (see Fig. 9.1, right-hand side).

The numerous interactions that take place during face-to-face decision making may be classified as either non-verbal or verbal communication. Although non-verbal communication is important, the focus in this book is on verbal communication because it is upon words and numbers that evidence-based clinical decisions are made.

Verbal communication in face-to-face decision making comprises three elements:

1. information given by the clinician after a diagnosis has been made;
2. interpretation by the patient;
3. discussion between clinician and patient.

For a patient to exercise choice based on the available evidence, all three elements must occur.

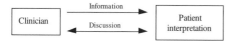

9.3 EVIDENCE-BASED PATIENT CHOICE

Communication with patients is a complicated topic that has many aspects, some of which are contentious, such as the issue of disclosure – how much should be revealed to patients, especially to those who are terminally ill?[1] In this book, the focus is on those aspects of communication that involve the provision, interpretation or discussion of evidence.

9.3.1 The provision of evidence-based information

Steps in the provision of evidence-based information to a patient include:

- finding all the available research evidence using the best possible searching techniques;

- appraising that research evidence to identify the best evidence available.

A systematic appraisal of the best evidence available includes the following calculations:

- the probability that the patient will benefit;
- the magnitude of any benefit;
- the probability that the patient will suffer adverse effects of treatment;
- the magnitude of any adverse effects.

However, it is possible that clinical ignorance might impede the delivery of effective care (see Box 9.1). Clinicians are not always aware of the best evidence available. In a study in which doctors' beliefs about the treatment of high blood pressure were compared with the effective treatment as based on the best evidence available,[2] it was found that doctors thought treatment should be commenced at a level of blood pressure that increased with the age of the patient whereas the evidence is that treatment is indicated at lower levels of blood pressure the older the patient (Fig. 9.2).

Even if a clinician is aware of the best evidence available, it may not be in a form that is relevant to the individual patient currently under care. When giving evidence-based information to a patient, the clinician must present that information in a form which patients will find useful. For example, in one study in which patients chose the therapy for lung cancer, it was found that patients would prefer it if the results were expressed in terms of life expectancy rather than in terms of the probability of surviving.[3]

Moreover, research indicates that doctors tend to emphasise the benefits rather than the adverse effects of treatment, as this harrowing account of a person treated for myeloid leukaemia illustrates.[4]

Box 9.1 Causes of clinical ignorance

- There may be no knowledge to know.
- There may be knowledge not known to the clinician.
- There may be knowledge known to the clinician, but that knowledge does not allow the clinician to assess the probabilities of the outcomes of the different options that face the clinician and the patient.

'We were told that the condition was serious, but in 50% of cases people were cured. When it was discovered there were sideroblasts the success rate was reduced to 25%. It was not until the second course of chemotherapy that the head of the department, B, saw Jeffrey and said that only 15% of patients can be treated successfully and for someone of Jeffrey's age a remission was impossible.'

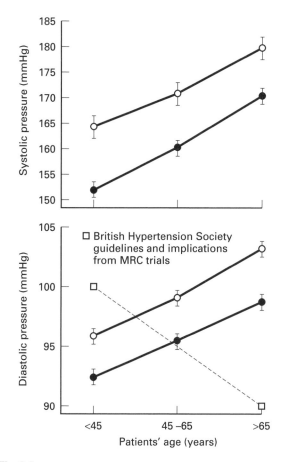

Fig. 9.2
Lowest systolic and diastolic blood pressure at which 125 general practitioners would define (●—●) and treat (○—○) hypertension. Values are means (95% confidence intervals); MRC = Medical Research Council (Source: Dickerson and Brown[2], with permission, BMJ Publishing Group)

When patients are given evidence, their preferences may change. In one study of people aged between 60 and 99 years who were asked if they wished to receive cardiopulmonary resuscitation (CPR), 41% said yes initially; when they were apprised of the evidence and realised that survival after CPR was lower than their expectations, the proportion of those wishing to receive it dropped to 22%.[5]

9.3.1.1   The power of the media

Clinicians are not the only source of evidence-based information for patients. The pharmaceutical industry sometimes uses the media to give evidence directly to patients. In 1991, for example, the results of one study showed that a new drug for high blood pressure had less of an effect on a patient's metabolism than the traditional treatment. The company that manufactured the drug immediately called a press conference and received front-page coverage in the *New York Times* and many other newspapers. Although no evidence on outcomes was presented, only that on intermediate variables such as the level of insulin sensitivity, patients were targeted directly with success.[6]

9.3.1.2   Evidence-based information about the process of care

The introduction of a new drug is usually easy; the means of administration will probably not differ from those of established drugs and therefore it is more likely to be acceptable to patients. In contrast, the introduction of a new operation is much more difficult; patients may want evidence about the skill of the operator. There are two inter-related questions the patient may ask: 'Should I have this operation?' and, if the answer is in the affirmative, 'Whom should I ask to perform this operation?' A patient's decision about whether to have an operation is usually determined by the level of confidence the patient has in a particular operator. This is wise because the evidence on which a clinician's advice is based is derived from trials in which high-quality professionals work within stringent criteria on a carefully defined and often relatively healthy subset of patients.

In this situation, a patient can ask for evidence about those characteristics of the process of care that have been demonstrated as leading to good outcomes. For example, any US patient considering laparoscopic cholecystectomy is advised by Nenner et al[7] to ask the questions shown in Box 9.2.

Box 9.2 (Source: Nenner et al[7])

- Is the surgeon board-certified?
- Does the surgeon have hospital privileges to do open cholecystectomy?
- Was the surgeon formally trained in a recognized program in laparoscopic cholecystectomy?
- How many laparoscopic cholecystectomies did he or she do and what were the frequency and types of complications?

9.3.2 Interpretation

Once a patient has been given the information, s/he has to interpret it, and may require time for reflection. The provision of written information (patient leaflets) can be used to support the verbal communication. Such leaflets can be used to give a clear indication of the strength of the evidence (see Fig. 9.3), for instance, by highlighting which statements are supported by research and which by opinion or anecdote.

A patient will seek to interpret the information in two ways.

1. How the evidence provided applies to his/her particular case: this is difficult for a patient, who may need guidance. It is the responsibility of the clinician to assess the relevance of the evidence to the particular patient who is consulting.
2. How the outcomes, good and bad, sit within the context of his/her values. For example, a patient who has deep vein thrombosis and is offered treatment needs to weigh up two risks:

   - that of death during treatment;
   - that of experiencing complications if treatment is refused.

In general, patients are more averse to the risks of serious side-effects than clinicians and, using decision analysis techniques, it is possible to delineate these values. In one study, all patients suspected of having venous thrombosis preferred to follow a course in which the risk of an early death from treatment was reduced rather than a course in which the risk of long-term complication from the disease was reduced.[8]

1. PRIMARY CARE MANAGEMENT OF STROKE IN THE COMMUNITY

❏ Aims

The guidelines# aim to improve the quality of stroke care by providing recommendations that are both scientifically valid and helpful in clinical practice for professionals caring for stroke patients in the community. They are consistent with the available scientific evidence [E] (at least one good randomised controlled trial) or, without such evidence, best clinical judgement [C]. A detailed systematic review of the literature can be obtained from Northamptonshire Health Authority.[1] Possible points for audit are indicated [AQ].

♦ Transient ischaemic attack (TIAs) will be discussed in relation to stroke prevention. The management of subarachnoid haemorrhage is not covered as it is clinically often regarded as a separate entity.

1. BLAIS, M.J. (1994) GRiP. *Using the evidence, Literature Review: Stroke.* Northampton: Northamptonshire Health Authority.

❏ How should patients / carers be supported?   [C]

(Please refer to guidelines on 'Stroke Rehabilitation and Aftercare following Hospitalisation' (no. 3)).

❏ Primary prevention   [E] [C] [AQ]

♦ Prevention must concentrate on the management of multiple risk factors:

➢ *Hypertension* (affected by diet, obesity, inadequate physical activity, excess alcohol, etc).

All patients should be given non-pharmalogical advice

• Reduce energy intake
• Reduce salt intake
• Avoid high saturated fat intake
• Avoid excessive alcohol
• Stop smoking
• Take regular exercise

#2. *Management of Stroke in Hospitals*
 3. *Stroke Rehabilitation and Aftercare Following Hospitalisation*

Fig. 9.3
Northamptonshire stroke leaflet

➢ *Hypertension.* Overall thresholds for intervention with drugs of ≥ 90 mm Hg, diastolic BP, and ≥ 160 mm Hg systolic BP are accepted, but with subgroups, e.g. younger age without coexisting risk factors, older age > 80 years, observation is indicated. *(Please refer to interim recommendations produced by the 'Second Working Party of the British Hypertension Society' for further details.)*

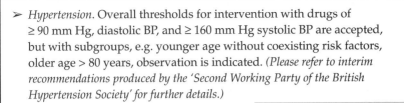

Thresholds of diastolic BP for intervention with drugs in younger patients

- ≥ 100 mm Hg – Treat
- 90–99 mm Hg – dependent on additional factors

Elderly patients

- Benefit from drug treatment
- Threshold ≥ 160 mm Hg systolic BP or ≥ 90 mm Hg diastolic BP, or both

○ Repeated measurement

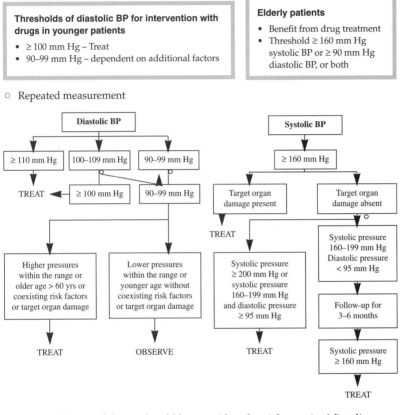

◆ Newer classes of drugs should be considered as 'alternative' first line agents when diuretics and β blockers are contraindicated or ineffective or when side effects occur.

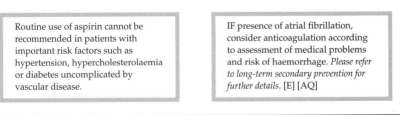

Routine use of aspirin cannot be recommended in patients with important risk factors such as hypertension, hypercholesterolaemia or diabetes uncomplicated by vascular disease.

IF presence of atrial fibrillation, consider anticoagulation according to assessment of medical problems and risk of haemorrhage. *Please refer to long-term secondary prevention for further details.* [E] [AQ]

9.3.3 Discussion

The quality of a discussion between clinician and patient is determined not by the quality of the evidence or the patient's knowledge of medical terms but primarily by the relationship between clinician and patient. If a patient feels powerless, the discussion will be stilted, inconclusive and unsatisfactory. If a patient feels empowered to participate with the clinician in decision making, a satisfactory discussion will take place.

9.3.4 Doctors: witch doctors or scientists?

Dear Reader,

Empathise with the eminent American surgeon and his son, who was also prominent in gastroenterology. The eminent surgeon developed stomach cancer. Father and son searched and appraised the literature: what was the best course of action? They went to see expert after expert. Each expert gave different advice or behaved so cautiously that they merely restated the evidence and said that it was inconclusive. Weary and dispirited, the son said to the last expert, 'What more do we need to get a good decision?' To which the expert replied, 'You need a good doctor'.

Commentary

Throughout most of this book, it has been argued that there is a need for a more scientific, evidence-based approach to decision making. However, there are situations in which clinical decisions are not clearcut, in fact only a small proportion ever are; as such, the relationship between clinician and patient is of central importance in decision taking. Although evidence is influential in decision making, in decision taking the fears, anxieties and values of the patient may predominate.

Although patients do want to be treated as rational beings, offered evidence, helped to assess the various options and left to take the decision, this model does not take account of the effect of an important element of any consultation, that of anxiety. Anxiety may be felt by both the clinician and the patient. Patients can be anxious about many aspects of illness and disease, such as the diagnosis, when it is unknown, or the treatment options and outcomes when it is.

Anthropologists have defined magic as an intervention designed to reduce anxiety in times of uncertainty; a rain dance does not bring rain but it does reduce anxiety during the wait. Witch doctors use only magic, although they can proffer what they may call 'evidence': for example, rain did fall after the rain dance. A witch doctor's role, therefore, is not to cure disease but to minimise anxiety in times of uncertainty.

Clinicians do use certain techniques to control patient anxiety, either consciously or unconsciously. One technique is to appear to be more certain, or to state or imply that the evidence of effectiveness is certain when, as is usually the case, it indicates only a probability of success. This is done with the best of intentions. It can be argued that the patient should have full disclosure of the evidence, as they would expect from a lawyer or a television engineer. Indeed, one speaker at a conference on bioethics in the USA said, 'I trust my lawyer more than I trust my doctor', meaning that she trusted the lawyer to tell her all the options and execute the one she chose, whereas she would not have this confidence in her doctors if she were terminally ill.

In a survey in the USA in 1982,[1] it was found that:

- 85% of Americans wanted a realistic estimate of 'how long they had to live if their type of cancer' usually leads to death in less than a year;
- only 41% of physicians if asked by a patient with 'a fully confirmed diagnosis of lung cancer at an advanced stage' would give either a straight statistical prognosis (13%) or 'say that you can't tell how long the patient might live but stress that in most cases people lived no longer than a year' (28%).

Some patients do want the clinician to deal with their anxiety, and look for reassurance and comfort; in fact, they require both a witch doctor and a doctor in the same consultation and in one and the same person.

Owing in part to the fear of litigation, clinicians are now more open and frank, particularly with patients who have a severe illness where a decision to proceed with treatment may expose the patient to interventions that have major side-effects but carry little prospect of cure. It is most common for this type of decision to be faced when there is a choice between further treatment for a malignancy or palliative care.

However, there is usually a dilemma associated with almost every clinical decision, not simply that associated with the choice between palliative care and interventions that have a low probability of success and a high risk of side-effects. Patients have to make decisions about whether to choose treatment A or treatment B, e.g. mastectomy or breast-conserving treatment (lumpectomy), or about whether to opt for preventive intervention or risk acceptance, e.g. treatment for high blood pressure or no action.

In one study of decisions made between two types of treatment, the association between being offered a choice of treatment and a patient being anxious or depressed after treatment was investigated. No difference was found in the prevalence of anxiety and depression between the patients who had been offered a choice of treatment and those to whom a firm recommendation had been made about a treatment option.[9] What is striking about this result is that it is impossible to generalise about patients and their preferences. For example, of the 62 women offered choice, eight refused to choose, whereas a proportion of patients who were not offered choice expressed a wish for more autonomy.

References

1. ANNAS, G.J. (1994) *Informed consent, cancer and truth in prognosis* . New Eng. J. Med. 330: 223–5.
2. DICKERSON, J.E.C. and BROWN, M.J. (1995) *Influence of age on general practitioners' definition and treatment of hypertension.* Br. Med. J. 310: 574.
3. McNEIL, B.J., PAUKER, S.G., SOX, H.C. and TVERSKY, A. (1982) *On the elicitation of preferences for alternative therapies.* New Eng. J. Med. 306: 1259–62.
4. ANONYMOUS (1994) *Dying for palliative care.* Br. Med. J. 309: 1696–9.
5. MURPHY, D.J., BURROWS, D., SANTILLI, S. et al. (1994) *The influence of the probability of survival on patients' preferences regarding cardiopulmonary resuscitation.* New Eng. J. Med. 330: 565–9.
6. MOSER, M., BLAUFOX, M.D., FRIES, E. et al. (1991) *Who really determines your patients' prescriptions?* JAMA 265: 498–500.
7. NENNER, R.P., IMPERATO, P.J. and WILL, T.O. (1994) *Questions patients should ask about laparoscopic cholecystectomy [Letter].* Ann. Intern. Med. 120: 443.
8. O'MEARA, J.J., MCNUTT, R.A., EVANS, A.T. et al. (1994) *A decision analysis of streptokinase plus heparin as compared with heparin alone for deep-vein thrombosis.* New Eng. J. Med. 330: 1864–9.
9. FALLOWFIELD, L.J., HALL, A., MAGUIRE, P. et al. (1994) *Psychological effects of being offered choice of surgery for breast cancer.* Br. Med. J. 309: 448.

9.4 EVIDENCE-BASED CLINICAL PRACTICE

Evidence-based clinical practice is the conscientious, explicit and judicious use of current best evidence when making decisions about individual patients.

The evidence-based practitioner should be using all the skills and resources described in this book to facilitate the process of clinical decision making. The use of the adjective 'judicious' signifies that the clinician must take into account a patient's condition, values and circumstances: evidence-based clinical practice is not cookbook medicine.[1] In evidence-based clinical practice, a clinician must link the evidence to the other activities that promote the exercise of evidence-based patient choice (see Fig. 9.4).

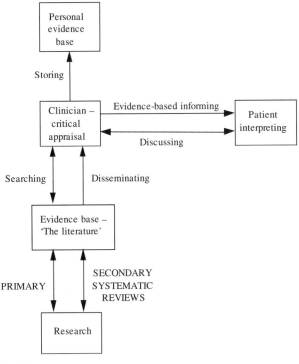

Fig. 9.4

Table 9.1

Evidence status	% of total patients			
	General medicine[2]	Psychiatry[3]	Surgery[4]	
			Elective	Emergency
Evidence from good-quality RCTs	53	65*	36	14
Convincing non-experimental evidence	29		57	70
Interventions without substantial evidence	18	35	7	16

*Evidence from RCTs and systematic reviews.

Contrary to the widely held belief that only 15–20% of clinical practice is based on good research, the evidence from general medicine,[2] psychiatry[3] and general surgery[4] is that the majority of patients are treated on the basis of good evidence (Table 9.1; see Table 7.3 for the evidence base for consultations in general practice).

There are, however, important failures in clinical decision making:

- ineffective interventions are introduced;
- interventions that do more harm than good are introduced;
- interventions that do more good than harm are not introduced;
- interventions that are ineffective or do more harm than good are not discontinued.

When considering the reasons why these failures happen, it is helpful to remember the three factors that drive clinical practice:

$$P = \frac{M \times C}{B}$$

Performance (P) is directly related to a professional's competence (C) and motivation (M) and inversely related to the barriers (B) that the professional has to overcome. There is no evidence that clinicians lack motivation, but some skills (competence) need to be improved and many barriers need to be removed.

Of those factors that contribute to the existence of barriers, some are external (Table 9.2), over which clinicians have very little control, and others are internal (Table 9.3), over which clinicians can exert an influence.

Table 9.2

External causes	Solutions outwith the power of clinicians
Poor quality of research producing biased evidence	Better training of research workers and more stringent ethics committees
Studies too small to produce unequivocal results	Promotion of systematic reviews
Unpublished research unavailable to clinicians	Publication of all research findings by pharmaceutical companies
Publication bias towards positive findings	Prevention of publication bias
Articles that cannot be found because of inadequate indexing	Better indexing
Failure of research workers to present evidence in forms useful to clinicians	Tougher action by journal editors
Inaccessible libraries	Extension of the World Wide Web to all clinicians

Table 9.3

Internal causes even a busy clinician can modify	Solutions for the busy clinician
Out-of-date textbooks	Don't read textbooks for guidance on therapy
Biased editorials and reviews	Don't read editorials and reviews for guidance on therapy except Cochrane and DARE reviews (see Appendix I)
Too much primary research (the average clinician needs to read 19 articles a day to keep up)	Read good-quality reviews rather than primary research
Reviews difficult to find	Improve searching skills (Sections 4.3.2 and 8.1)
Inability to spot flaws in research	Improve appraisal skills (Sections 4.3.3 and 8.2)
Difficulty in retrieving evidence identified as useful	Develop skills to use reference management software (Section 8.3).
Translating the data about groups of patients in research papers into information relevant to an individual patient	Develop/improve understanding of baseline risk and NNT (Section 6.3.3.1) and ability to explain how research results apply to an individual patient (Section 9.3.1)[5-7]
Insufficient time	Be more discerning about what to read by developing a good scanning strategy (Box 4.1, p 65)

References

1. SACKETT, D.L., ROSENBERG, W.M.C., GRAY, J.A.M. et al. (1996) *Evidence-based medicine: what it is and what it isn't [Editorial].* Br. Med. J. 312: 71–2.
2. ELLIS, J., MULLIGAN, I., ROWE, J. and SACKETT, D.L. (1995) *In-patient general medicine is evidence based.* Lancet 346: 407–10.
3. GEDDES, J., GAME, D., JENKINS, N.E., PETERSON, L.A., PORRINGER, G.R. and SACKETT, D.L. *What proportion of primary psychiatric interventions are based on randomised evidence?* Quality in Health Care. In Press.
4. McCULLOCH, P. and SACKETT, D.L. *Evidence-based surgery: the importance of quality.* In press.
5. GUYATT, G.H., COOK, D.J. and JAESCHKE, R. (1995) *How should clinicians use the results of randomized trials?* ACP Journal Club Jan–Feb: 122(1): A12–3.

6. GUYATT, H.G., COOK, D.J. and JAESCHKE, R. (1995) *Applying the findings of clinical trials to individual patients [Editorial].* ACP Journal Club Mar–Apr: 122(2): A12–3.
7. GLASZIOU, P.P. and IRWIG, L.M. (1995) *An evidence based approach to individualising treatment.* Br. Med. J. 311: 1356–9.

9.5   ACCELERATING CHANGE IN CLINICAL PRACTICE

Clinical practice is changing all the time. Over the last two decades, the medical profession as a whole has performed well in discarding ineffective therapies and adopting effective ones. However, in the current economic climate, the evolution of clinical practice must be telescoped. At present, the process of evolution is marked by the following characteristics:

* overenthusiastic adoption of interventions of unproven efficacy or even proven ineffectiveness;
* failure to adopt interventions that do more good than harm at a reasonable cost;
* continuing to offer interventions or services demonstrated to be ineffective;
* adoption of interventions without adequate preparation such that the benefits demonstrated in a research setting cannot be reproduced in the ordinary service setting;
* wide variation in the rates at which interventions are adopted or discarded.

9.5.1   Educate to influence

Within the numerous RCTs of different interventions designed to improve clinical practice, patient outcome has been taken as the end-point and not a professional's knowledge or level of skill. The results of such trials, which measure the outcomes that matter most to patients, should be of interest to educators and those who provide funds for education.

In continuing medical education, the following interventions have not been shown to be effective:

* standard lectures;
* the provision of knowledge alone;
* written information.

There is also evidence that for clinicians some form of educational needs assessment and setting of learning objectives is a necessary precursor to identify the topics about which an individual needs to learn.[1] Formal training can improve performance with respect to these topics. However, for those topics individuals wish to study, knowledge base and performance improves irrespective of training.

In a systematic review of 150 RCTs of different methods of continuing medical education,[2] the following interventions were found to be effective in changing behaviour.

- Mini-sabbaticals – allowing clinicians to go and work in units practising high-quality evidence-based healthcare.
- Sensitive personalised feedback on an individual's performance, either in comparison with that of others or against explicit standards, as part of a learning process.
- Patient education.
- Computer-assisted decision making providing reminders and easy access to evidence-based guidelines and to knowledge itself.
- On-the-job training of practical skills.
- The use of opinion leaders or 'educational influentials', i.e. a colleague whose performance is respected.

It could be argued that these interventions will increase cost. However, it is also important to determine the cost of failing to offer such education and of the current level of expenditure on continuing professional education using techniques of unproven effectiveness.

9.5.2   Carrots or sticks?

Two schools of thought have culminated in a polarisation of views: there are those who believe in incentives (the carrot) and those who believe in disincentives (the stick) as a means of achieving change. An interesting permutation that one commentator advocated was to hit people with the carrot!

The evidence of whether a carrot or a stick is more effective is difficult to interpret, in part because of the problem in defining what constitutes a carrot and what constitutes a stick. The introduction of incentive payments for cervical screening for general practitioners played a part in increasing the coverage of cervical screening. Was the money a carrot or was the threat of a drop in income a stick? Financial incentives are difficult to manage and it is easy for perverse incentives to be introduced into any system. The simplest system in which to operate evidence-based healthcare is one in which physicians are salaried and receive no financial reward for increased volume or intensity of care, as George Bernard Shaw so elegantly articulated.

'It is not the fault of our doctors that the medical service of the community, as at present provided for, is a murderous absurdity. That any sane nation, having observed that you could provide for the supply of bread by giving bakers a pecuniary interest in baking for you, should go on to give a surgeon a pecuniary interest in cutting off your leg, is enough to make one despair of political humanity. But that is precisely what we have done. And the more appalling the mutilation, the more the mutilator is paid. He who corrects the ingrowing toe-nail receives a few shillings: he who cuts your inside out receives hundreds of guineas, except when he does it to a poor person for practice.'

From 'Preface on Doctors', in *The Doctor's Dilemma*, 1911

If healthcare is delivered within a fee-based service, for example, in a private insurance scheme, it is easy to influence practice by stopping paying for a particular procedure. The response is usually marked and quick.

In systems in which finance is not a strong motivator, external pressures can be applied through the use of guidelines and other aspects of 'managed care' (Section 7.3.2). However, even in the preparation of guidelines, external pressures, whether as carrots or sticks, are relatively ineffective. In an evaluation of guidelines as a means of influencing clinical practice,[3] a wide variation was found ranging from nationally produced guidelines, which are evidence-based but relatively ineffective, to locally produced guidelines, in which local practitioners have been involved, which can be effective but may also be unscientific.

When developing a set of guidelines, the aim should be to ensure that the right evidence base is available and that it is used to develop clinical policies locally (Fig. 9.5). Although such policies can be expressed within guidelines or protocols, it is important that they are owned by those whom it is sought to influence. It is said that Mary Baker's famous cake mixes were not selling well until the powdered egg was withdrawn and customers were required to break an egg into the mixture. The evidence suggests the same is true when making clinical policies.[3]

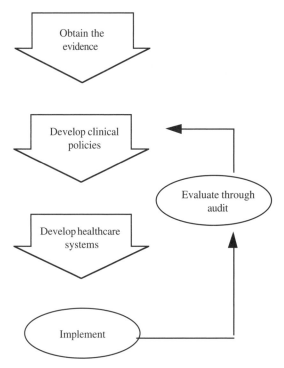

Fig. 9.5
From research to implementation and audit

9.5.3 Growing carrots

The use of the simplistic carrot and stick metaphor implies that the only change that needs to take place is a change in clinical practice. However, to take such a narrow focus will have only a limited impact, even if all of the interventions shown to be effective in changing clinical practice are used.

Change is happening at an exponential rate, thereby increasing the pressure on professionals within a context of decreasing availability of resources. In this situation, it is essential to appreciate the wider context,[4] otherwise it will not be possible to overcome what has been called 'the subtle sabotage of withheld enthusiasm'.[5]

The most important step in facilitating change is to ensure that professionals want to change. The most effective way of encouraging professionals to change is to help them see evidence-based decision making not as a management imperative but as an intellectual challenge. It is much more effective to stimulate professionals to grow their own carrots than to force them into behaving like donkeys, enticed by a carrot dangling in front and threatened by a stick held behind.

References

1. SIBLEY, J.C., SACKETT, D.L., NEUFELD, V.R. et al. (1982) *A randomized trial of continuing medical education.* New Eng. J. Med. 302: 511.
2. DAVIS. D.A., THOMSON, M.A., OXMAN, A.D. and HAYNES, B.P. (1995) *Changing physicians' performance.* JAMA 274: 700–5.
3. GRIMSHAW, J.M. and RUSSELL, I.T. (1993) *Effect of clinical guidelines on medical practice: a systematic review of rigorous evaluations.* Lancet 342: 1317–22.
4. BACKER, T.E. (1995) *Integrating behavioral and systems strategies to change clinical practice.* J. Quality Improvement 21: 351–3.
5. KAEGI, L. (1993) *Using guidelines to change clinical behavior: dissemination through Area Health Centers and Geriatric Education Centers.* Quality Review Bulletin May: 165–9.

SOURCES OF EVIDENCE

A. PUBLISHED EVIDENCE

Evidence is available in two main forms.

1. Reviews of primary research: of variable quality. However, for some reviews, known as systematic reviews, the methods that were used to identify, appraise and analyse the primary research are stated explicitly so that readers can decide for themselves how strong the evidence is. Systematic reviews are written for decision makers, who are users of research, and also for researchers because every project for which new data is to be collected, i.e. 'primary research', should be preceded by a systematic review of what is known and be concluded by incorporating that new data into a revised systematic review. This procedure is not always followed, although examples of this approach are beginning to appear in the literature.[1]

   Where to search for reviews: MEDLINE (see A.4), EMBASE (see A.5) and other databases, using the searching strategies described in Appendix II.

   Warning: reviews, like textbooks, may be biased and misleading.

   Solution: use The Cochrane Library (see A.1) and also search other good-quality reviews (see A.2).

2. Primary research: usually published in scientific journals; of variable quality and written primarily by researchers for other researchers. As the primary research base is enormous and is increasing rapidly, the primary literature should be accessed only after attempts have been made to find the evidence needed from systematic reviews.

   Where to search: databases such as MEDLINE (see A.4) and EMBASE (see A.5).

Warning: the problems inherent with electronic databases (see Chapter 4) mean that searching the primary research literature is not necessarily productive in terms of the comprehensiveness of the evidence collected.

Solution: search subject specialist databases (see A.6)

A.1   The Cochrane Library

The Cochrane Library is a regularly updated electronic library designed to provide the evidence needed for healthcare decision making. It was launched in April 1995 under the name the Cochrane Database of Systematic Reviews, but it has now been re-named to reflect the inclusion of further important related databases.
The Cochrane Library now contains:

- the Cochrane Database of Systematic Reviews (CDSR);
- the York Database of Abstracts of Reviews of Effectiveness (DARE);
- the Cochrane Controlled Trials Register (CCTR);
- the Cochrane Review Methodology Database (CRMD)
  The following specifications are required to run
  The Cochrane Library: PC with 386SX processor or higher, both with 4 MB RAM minimum and a hard disk with at least 15 MB of free space. To subscribe to The Cochrane Library, contact: Update Software, PO Box 696, Oxford OX2 7YX; tel: (+44)-1865-513902; fax: (+44)-1865-516918; email: update@cochrane.co.uk; URL: http://update.cochrane.co.uk/info

A.1.1   The Cochrane Database of Systematic Reviews (CDSR)

- A rapidly growing collection of regularly updated systematic reviews of the effects of healthcare.
- Prepared by contributors to the Cochrane Collaboration (see Box A.I.1), an international network of individuals committed to 'preparing, maintaining and disseminating systematic reviews of the effects of healthcare'.
- Nearly 100 Cochrane reviews are currently available in the areas of pregnancy and childbirth, subfertility, stroke, schizophrenia, and parasitic diseases. In addition, there are 94 protocols in the areas of acute respiratory infections, airways, diabetes, musculoskeletal injuries, neonatal care, and peripheral vascular diseases.

- New reviews will be added with each issue of The Cochrane Library, so that eventually all areas of healthcare will be covered.

The systematic reviews are prepared, and maintained, according to the standards set out in Section 6 of The Cochrane Collaboration Handbook. They are based on hand searching of journals and prepared by personnel who will also be responsible for identifying and incorporating new evidence as it becomes available.

Box A.I.1   The Cochrane Collaboration

'The Cochrane Collaboration is an enterprise that rivals the Human Genome Project in its potential implications for modern medicine.'[2]

The Cochrane Collaboration is an international research initiative set up to produce, maintain and disseminate systematic reviews of the evidence about the prevention and treatment or control of health problems.

The need for the Cochrane Collaboration was identified because:

- no decision maker can stay abreast of the scientific literature;
- textbooks quickly become out-of-date, particularly with respect to treatment regimens;[3]
- editorials, and reviews in which there is no explicit statement of the methods of searching, the criteria for inclusion and exclusion, and the analytical techniques (i.e. they are not systematic), are biased and unreliable;[4]
- MEDLINE and EMBASE cover less than half of the world's journals;
- of the randomised trials in MEDLINE, only about half can be found by an expert searcher, and an experienced clinical searcher will find only half the trials that an expert searcher can find;[5]
- even when trials can be found, they are often of inadequate power and are biased towards the reporting of positive findings;[6, 7]
- even when reviews are systematic and of high quality, they quickly become out-of-date.

The two main types of organisational unit of the Cochrane Collaboration are:

- Cochrane Centres;
- Collaborative Review Groups.

By 1997, there will be more than ten Cochrane Centres around the world and a growing number of Collaborative Review Groups.

Address: The UK Cochrane Centre, NHS R&D Programme, Summertown Pavilion, Middle Way, Oxford OX2 7LG; tel (+44)-1865-516300; fax (+44)-1865-516311; email: general@cochrane.co.uk; URL: http://hiru.mcmaster.ca/cochrane/

A.1.2   The York Database of Abstracts of Reviews of Effectiveness (DARE)

Complementing the information on CDSR, DARE provides:

- structured abstracts of over 100 further good-quality systematic reviews from around the world, all of which have been quality filtered by reviewers at the NHS Centre for Reviews and Dissemination at the University of York, England (see Box A.I.2);
- briefer records of reviews which may be useful for background information;
- abstracts of reports of health technology agencies worldwide;
- abstracts of reviews produced by the *American College of Physicians (ACP) Journal Club* up to 1995.

The reviews in this database must meet all of the following criteria:

- be reports of reviews completed within the last five years;
- be relevant to assessing the effects of healthcare;
- be based on a thorough search for potentially eligible studies, which is documented;
- be governed by explicit criteria for including studies in the review;
- contain a summary of the studies included, presented either as a summary table of study characteristics or a summary table or graph of individual study results.

Box A.I.2   The NHS Centre for Reviews and Dissemination (NHS CRD)

The CRD is a facility commissioned by the NHS Research and Development Division. The aim of the CRD is to identify and review the results of good-quality health research and to disseminate the findings to decision makers within the NHS and to consumers of health services. The reviews cover:

- the effectiveness of care for particular conditions;
- the effectiveness of health technologies;
- evidence on efficient methods of organising and delivering particular types of healthcare.

Address: University of York, York, YO1 5DD; email: revdis@york.ac.uk.
URL: http://www.york.ac.uk/inst/crd/dissem.htm

A.1.3   The Cochrane Controlled Trials Register (CCTR)

A bibliography of over 100 000 controlled trials identified by contributors to the Cochrane Collaboration and others, including many trials not currently listed in MEDLINE or other bibliographic databases.

N.B. The complete CCTR is only available on the CD ROM version of The Cochrane Library. The disk-based version includes only the 1995 and 1996 trials from the CCTR (over 12 000).

A.1.4   The Cochrane Review Methodology Database (CRMD)

A bibliography of articles on the science of research synthesis and on practical aspects of preparing systematic reviews. An invaluable source of information on RCTs, and the strengths and weaknesses of systematic reviews.

A.2   NHS CRD Publications

A.2.1   CRD Reports

1. Which way forward for the care of critically ill children?
2. Relationship between volume and quality of health care: a review of the literature.
3. Review of the research on the effectiveness of health service interventions to reduce variations in health.
4. Undertaking systematic reviews of research on effectiveness. CRD Guidelines for those carrying out or commissioning reviews.
5. Ethnicity and health: reviews of literature and guidance for purchasers in the areas of cardiovascular disease, mental health and haemoglobinopathies.

To order CRD Reports, contact CRD Publications:
tel: (+44)-1904-433648.

A.2.2   Effectiveness Matters

This series provides updates on the effectiveness of important health interventions for practitioners and decision makers in the NHS.

1. Aspirin and myocardial infarction
2. *Helicobacter pylori* and peptic ulcer

Effectiveness Matters is a free publication available on subscription. To subscribe, contact CRD Publications: tel: (+44)-1904-433648.

A.2.3   Effective Health Care

Effective Health Care is a bimonthly bulletin for decision makers in which the effectiveness of a variety of healthcare interventions is examined, based on a systematic review and synthesis of research on clinical effectiveness, cost-effectiveness and acceptability. Reviews are carried out by a research team using established methodological guidelines, with advice from expert consultants for each topic.

Volume 1
1. Screening for osteoporosis to prevent fractures
2. Stroke rehabilitation
3. The management of subfertility
4. The treatment of persistent glue ear in children
5. The treatment of depression in primary care
6. Cholesterol: screening and treatment
7. Brief interventions and alcohol abuse
8. Implementing clinical practice guidelines
9. Management of menorrhagia

Volume 2
1. The prevention and treatment of pressure sores
2. Benign prostatic hyperplasia: treatment for lower urinary tract symptoms in older men
3. Management of cataract
4. Preventing falls and subsequent injury in older people
5. Preventing unintentional injuries in children and young adolescents

The bulletin is produced by the CRD with the Nuffield Institute for Health at the University of Leeds, and published by Churchill Livingstone.

All orders and enquiries regarding subscriptions should be addressed to: Churchill Livingstone Subscriptions Department, P.O. Box 77, Fourth Avenue, Harlow, CM19 5BQ; tel: (+44)-1279-623924; fax: (+44)-1279-639609.

These reviews are systematic because they are written to standards set out in the Centre's *Guidelines for those carrying out or commissioning reviews*.[8] These guidelines are excellent, pulling together the skills of writing and presenting systematic reviews.

A.3 Other good-quality reviews

There are other sources of reviewed evidence which,
although they do not meet the full Cochrane Collaboration
or NHS CRD standards, can be recommended.

A.3.1 DEC Reports from the Wessex Institute of Public Health

These reports are technology assessments prepared initially
for the Development and Evaluation Committee of the
Wessex Regional Health Authority. They can be found on the
Web page of the South and West Regional R&D Programme
of the NHS: URL: http://cochrane.epi.bris.ac.uk/rd/

A.3.2 Systematic reviews from the NHS R&D Programme

In the UK, the NHS R&D Programme has a number of
national Priority Research Programmes (see Box A.I.3).
   Within each programme, systematic reviews are produced
in addition to 'primary research'. Information about
the reviews that have been commissioned can be found
at this Web site:
URL: http://libsun1.jr2.ox.ac.uk/a-ordd/index.htm

Box A.I.3 Priority research programmes in the UK NHS R&D Strategy

Mental health programme
Cardiovascular disease and stroke programme
Physical and complex disabilities programme
Cancer programme
Primary and secondary care interface programme
Research into the effective implementation of research findings
Mother and child health
Asthma management programme
Health technology assessment programme
The policy research programme

A.3.3   Clinical Standards Advisory Group reports

Reports published by the Clinical Standards Advisory Group are reviews of variations in the quality and effectiveness of healthcare throughout England.

- Access to and availability of specialist services. London: HMSO; 1993; ISBN: 0 11 321 596 7
- Back pain. London: HMSO; 1994; ISBN 0 11 321 887 7
- Childhood leukaemia: access and availability of specialist services. London: HMSO; 1993; ISBN: 0 11 321 598 3
- Coronary artery bypass grafting and coronary angioplasty: access to and availability of specialist services. London: HMSO; 1993; ISBN: 0 11 321 597 5
- Cystic fibrosis: access to and availability of specialist services. London: HMSO; 1993; ISBN: 0 11 321 600 9
- Dental general anaesthesia. London: HMSO; 1995; ISBN: 0 11 321 924 5
- Epidemiology review: the epidemiology and cost of back pain. London: HMSO; 1994; ISBN: 0 11 321 889 3
- Neonatal intensive care: access to and availability of specialist services. London: HMSO; 1993; ISBN: 0 11 321 599 1
- Schizophrenia: volume 1. London: HMSO; 1995; ISBN: 0 11 321 929 6
- Schizophrenia: volume II. London: HMSO; 1995; ISBN: 0 11 321 922 9
- Standards of clinical care for people with diabetes. London: HMSO; 1994; ISBN: 0 11 321 819 2
- Urgent and emergency admissions. London: HMSO; 1995; ISBN: 0 11 321 835 4
- Women in normal labour. London: HMSO; 1995; ISBN: 0 11 321 923 7
- Department of Health. Government response to the reports by the Clinical Standards Advisory Group on access to and availability of specialist services. London: Department of Health; 1993.

A.3.4   The epidemiologically based needs assessment reviews

This series of health care needs assessment reviews was developed out of the NHS Management Executive's (NHSME) District Health Authority project which was set up to clarify the components of the purchasing role. This role was seen to include:

- the need and demand for healthcare;
- an appraisal of service options;
- monitoring of services and health.

Twenty topics were selected against the following criteria:

- the 'burden of disease' (i.e. mortality and morbidity) and the financial implications for the health service;
- the scope for changing purchasing patterns in the future;
- the need to test the method used for needs assessment using a wide range of topics.

As such, these reviews provide guidance for purchasers about the incidence and prevalence of certain health problems and the effective means of tackling those problems on the basis of a review of the evidence. These reviews have now been published in the following format:

STEVENS, A. and RAFTERY, J. (Eds) (1994) *Health care needs assessment: the epidemiologically based needs assessment reviews.* Radcliffe Medical Publications, Oxford

Volume 1
- Introduction
- Diabetes mellitus
- Renal disease
- Stroke (acute cerebrovascular disease)
- Lower respiratory disease
- Coronary heart disease
- Colorectal cancer
- Cancer of the lung
- Total hip replacement
- Total knee replacement
- Cataract surgery

Volume 2
- Hernia repair
- Varicose vein treatments
- Prostatectomy for benign prostatic hyperplasia
- Mental illness
- Dementia
- Alcohol misuse
- Drug abuse
- People with learning difficulties
- Community child health services
- Family planning, abortion and fertility services
- Reflections and conclusions

A.4   MEDLINE

The National Library of Medicine's bibliographic database covers the international literature on biomedicine, including the allied health fields and the biological and physical sciences, the humanities, and information science as they relate to medicine and healthcare. Information is indexed from approximately 3700 journals worldwide. MEDLINE covers from 1966 to the present. Refer to Box A.I.4 for some useful term definitions from MEDLINE.

A.5   EMBASE

Elsevier Science's bibliographic database covers biomedical literature from 110 countries and has particular strengths in the areas of drugs and toxicology. EMBASE is the short form of the Excerpta Medica database, and has a strong coverage of European material. Information is indexed from approximately 3500 journals. EMBASE covers from 1974 to the present.

A.6   Subject specialist databases

A.6.1   Subject specialist bibliographic databases

There is a large number of specialised bibliographic databases; for example, on cancer or nursing and allied health disciplines. The librarian will be able to help you identify and find these.

A.6.1.1   HealthSTAR

HealthSTAR contains citations to the published literature on health services, technology, administration and research. It is focused on both the clinical and non-clinical aspects of healthcare delivery. The following topics are included: evaluation of patient outcomes; effectiveness of procedures, programmes, products, services and processes; administration and planning of health facilities, services and manpower; health insurance; health policy; health services research; health economics and financial management; laws and regulation; personnel administration; quality assurance; licensure; accreditation. HeathSTAR is produced co-operatively by the National Library of Medicine and the American Hospital Association. The database contains citations and abstracts when available to journal articles, monographs, technical reports, meeting abstracts and

papers, book chapters, government documents
and newspaper articles form 1975 to the present.
HealthSTAR is updated monthly.

Box A.I.4 Some useful term notes and/or definitions of terms from MEDLINE

Research design A plan for collecting and utilising data so that desired information
can be obtained with sufficient precision or so that an hypothesis can be tested
properly.

Clinical trials Pre-planned studies of the safety, efficacy or optimum dosage schedule
(if appropriate) of one or more diagnostic, therapeutic or prophylactic drugs, devices
or techniques, selected according to predetermined criteria of eligibility and observed
for predefined evidence of favourable and unfavourable effects. This concept
includes clinical trials conducted both in the US and in other countries.

Randomized controlled trials Clinical trials that involve at least one test treatment
and one control treatment, concurrent enrolment and follow-up of the test- and
control-treated groups, and in which the treatments to be administered are selected
by a random process, such as the use of a random-numbers table. Treatment
allocations using coin flips, odd–even numbers, patient social security numbers,
days of the week, medical record numbers, or other such pseudo- or quasi-random
processes, are not truly randomised and trials employing any of these techniques for
patient assignment are designated simply CONTROLLED CLINICAL TRIALS.

Random allocation A process involving chance used in therapeutic trials or other
research endeavour for allocating experimental subjects, human or animal, between
treatment and control groups, or among treatment groups. It may also apply to
experiments on inanimate objects.

Meta-analysis A quantitative method of combining the results of independent
studies (usually drawn from the published literature) and synthesising summaries
and conclusions which may be used to evaluate therapeutic effectiveness, plan new
studies, etc., with application chiefly in the areas of research and medicine.

Cohort studies Studies in which subsets of a defined population are identified.
These groups may or may not be exposed to factors hypothesised to influence the
probability of the occurrence of a particular disease or other outcome. Cohorts are
defined populations which, as a whole, are followed in an attempt to determine
distinguishing subgroup characteristics.

Case-control studies Studies which start with the identification of persons with a
disease of interest and a control (comparison, referent) group without the disease.
The relationship of an attribute to the disease is examined by comparing diseased
and non-diseased persons with regard to the frequency or levels of the attribute in
each group.

A.6.2 Journals of secondary publication

As most journals are published primarily for research workers, several journals of secondary publication have been originated.

The first of these was the *American College of Physicians (ACP) Journal Club*, which is published bimonthly. It provides detailed abstracts of high quality and relevant studies from over 20 top journals in the field of general medicine and allied specialties. Abstracts/studies are set out systematically: all the information is provided on one page, including a commentary. The last sentence of each commentary is made into the title of the article; the title is set in the present tense if the paper is a systematic review, and in the past tense if the paper is an RCT (the rationale behind this is that an RCT summarises what was found, whereas a systematic review summarises what is known).

Although the *ACP Journal Club* is published as a supplement to the *Annals of Internal Medicine*, it can be obtained separately. It is now also available on CD ROM; contact: Customer Service Center, American College of Physicians, Independence Mall West, Sixth Street at Race, Philadelphia, PA19106, USA.

A.6.2.1 Evidence-Based Medicine

This is a new journal, a complementary companion to the *ACP Journal Club*, covering not only general medicine but also obstetrics and gynaecology, psychiatry, surgery anaesthesia, paediatrics and general practice.

These two journals should be included in any scanning strategy, not only for the evidence they contain but also for the articles included about the research methods used and the concepts employed, such as absolute risk reduction and number needed to treat (NNT).

Other journals of secondary publication are being planned, the most important of which to readers of this book will be the *Journal of Evidence-Based Healthcare Policy and Management* (to be launched by Churchill Livingstone in 1997).

A.6.3 Registers of published research

It is also important to be alert to the publication of registers of published research. The *Register of Cost-Effectiveness Studies*, produced by the Economics and Operational Research Division of the Department of Health in 1994, is an excellent example of this type of register.

References

1. ISIS–1 COLLABORATIVE GROUP (1986) *Randomised trial of intravenous atenolol among 16, 027 cases of suspected acute myocardial infarction.* Lancet ii: 57–66.
2. NAYLOR, C.D. (1995) *Grey zones of clinical practice: some limits to evidence-based medicine.* Lancet 345: 840–2.
3. ANTMAN, E.M., LAU, J., KUPELNICK, B. et al. (1992) *A comparison of results of meta-analysis of randomized control trials and recommendations of clinical experts.* JAMA, 268: 240–8.
4. MOHER, D. and OLKIN, I. (1995) *Meta-analysis of randomized controlled trials. A concern for standards.* JAMA 274: 1962–4.
5. ADAMS, C.E., POWER, A., FREDERICK, K. and LEFEBVRE, C. (1994) *An investigation of the adequacy of MEDLINE searches for randomized controlled trials (RCTs) of the effects of mental health care.* Psychol. Med. 24: 741–8.
6. GØTZSCHE, P. (1989) *Methodology and overt and hidden bias in reports of 196 double-blind trials of nonsteroidal anti-inflammatory drugs in rheumatoid arthritis.* Controlled Clinical Trials 10: 31–56.
7. SCHULZ, K.F., CHALMERS, I., HAYES, R.J. and ALTMAN, D. (1995) *Empirical evidence of bias. Dimensions of methodological quality associated with estimates of treatment effects in controlled trials.* JAMA 273: 408–12.
8. DEEKS, J., GLANVILLE, J. and SHELDON, T. (1996) *Undertaking systematic reviews of effectiveness: Guidelines for those carrying out or commissioning reviews.* CRD Publications, York.

Further reading

CHALMERS, I. and ALTMAN, D.G. (1995) *Systematic Reviews.* BMJ Publications, London.

B.   UNPUBLISHED EVIDENCE: REGISTERS OF RESEARCH IN PROGRESS

It is very important to identify research in progress, such that one can complement the question 'What has been found out?' with the question 'What is being found out?'. There are two major registers of research in progress, each of which point to other specialised research registers.

B.1   The National Research Register

The National Research Register (NRR) is a register of research currently being funded by the Department of Health and NHS R&D Programme. It is available in all offices of the NHS R&D Programme; from 1997, it will be available in every healthcare library in the UK. Further information about the National Research Register can be obtained from the R&D Directorate at NHS Executive Headquarters, Quarry House, Quarry Hill, Leeds LS2 7UE; tel: (+44)-113-254-6187.

B.2 Database of current health services research (HSRProj)

This is a database of current health services research projects funded by government agencies and private foundations in the USA. It is an online facility provided by the US National Library of Medicine (NLM), and is produced jointly by the National Library of Medicine, the Association for Health Services Research, and the University of North Carolina at Chapel Hill. Its development is being co-ordinated by the National Information Center on Health Services Research and Health Care Technology. It is searchable using the NLM's Grateful Med Software.

The National Library of Medicine is one of the world's great knowledge treasuries; for information about the databases that are available from the NLM, consult the NLM's home page: URL: http://www.nlm.nih.gov

Address: National Library of Medicine, US Department of Health and Human Services, Public Health Service, National Institutes of Health, Bethesda, MD20894, USA.

Address: Association for Health Services Research, 1350 Connecticut Avenue, Suite 1100, Washington DC20036, USA.

SEARCHING

INTRODUCTION

Included in this appendix are two examples of search strategies prepared by the Cochrane Collaboration and included in The Cochrane Collaboration Handbook (for URL see p 223). As databases are enlarged or as new databases develop, search strategies must be altered. Good advice on searching for RCTs and systematic reviews, from which this information is abstracted, is given in The Cochrane Library (see Appendix I).

Further information on searching is provided at the World Wide Web site developed to support this book (URL: http://www.ihs.ox.ac.uk/ebh.html) and the companion volume by Sackett et al on evidence-based medicine, *Evidence-Based Medicine: How to Practice and Teach EBM* (URL: http://cebm.jr2.ox.ac.uk/dovs/toolbox.htm).

MEDLINE SEARCH STRATEGY FOR ASTHMA / AIR POLLUTANTS SYSTEMATIC REVIEWS

#1   explode 'AIR-POLLUTANTS, -ENVIRONMENTAL'/ all subheadings
#2   explode 'ASTHMA'/ all subheadings
#3   REVIEW-ACADEMIC in PT
#4   REVIEW-TUTORIAL in PT
#5   META-ANALYSIS in PT
#6   'META-ANALYSIS'
#7   (SYSTEMATIC* near REVIEW*) in TI
#8   (SYSTEMATIC* near REVIEW*) in AB
#9   (SYSTEMATIC* near OVERVIEW*) in TI
#10 (SYSTEMATIC* near OVERVIEW*) in AB
#11 META? ANALY* in TI
#12 META? ANALY* in AB
#13 #3 or #4 or #5 or #6 or #7 or #8 or #9 or #10 or #11 or #12
#14 (TG=ANIMAL) not (TG=HUMAN)
#15 #13 not #14
#16 #1 and #2 and #15

This strategy is based on a search strategy developed by Carol Lefebvre on behalf of the Cochrane Collaboration. The strategy is being developed further by the NHS Centre for Reviews and Dissemination at the University of York. An updated version can be viewed on the World Wide Web at: http://www.york.ac.uk/inst/crd/dissem.htm

MEDLINE SEARCH STRATEGY FOR ASTHMA / AIR POLLUTANTS RCTS

#1   explode 'AIR-POLLUTANTS, -ENVIRONMENTAL'/
     all subheadings
#2   explode 'ASTHMA'/ all subheadings
#3   RANDOMIZED CONTROLLED TRIAL in PT
#4   CONTROLLED CLINICAL TRIAL in PT
#5   'RANDOMIZED-CONTROLLED-TRIALS'/
     all subheadings
#6   'RANDOM-ALLOCATION'
#7   'DOUBLE-BLIND-METHOD'
#8   'SINGLE-BLIND-METHOD'
#9   #3 or #4 or #5 or #6 or #7 or #8
#10 CLINICAL TRIAL in PT
#11 explode 'CLINICAL-TRIALS'/ all subheadings
#12 (CLIN* near TRIAL*) in TI
#13 (CLIN* near TRIAL*) in AB
#14 (SINGL* or DOUBL* or TREBL* or TRIPL*) near
     (BLIND* or MASK*)
#15 (#14 in TI) or (#14 in AB)
#16 'PLACEBOS'/ all subheadings
#17 PLACEBO* in TI
#18 PLACEBO* in AB
#19 RANDOM* in TI
#20 RANDOM* in AB
#21 'RESEARCH-DESIGN'/ all subheadings
#22 VOLUNTEER* in TI
#23 VOLUNTEER* in AB
#24 #10 or #11 or #12 or #13 or #15 or #16 or #17 or #18
     or #19 or #20 or #21 or #22 or #23
#25 #9 or #24
#26 (TG=ANIMAL) not (TG=HUMAN)
#27 #25 not #26
#28 #1 and #2 and #27

This strategy is based on a search strategy developed by
Carol Lefebvre on behalf of the Cochrane Collaboration.
An updated version can be viewed on the World Wide Web
at: http://hiru.mcmaster.ca/cochrane/

APPRAISING

A. MORE DETAILED READING ON CRITICAL APPRAISAL

- MILNE, R. and CHAMBERS, L. (1993) *Assessing the scientific quality of review articles.* Epid. Commun. Hlth. 43: 169–70.

A.1 Users' Guides to the Medical Literature

The following series by the Evidence-Based Medicine Working Group is an extremely useful collection of articles.

- GUYATT, D.H. and RENNIE, D. (1993) *Users' Guides to the Medical Literature.* JAMA 270: 2096–7.
- OXMAN, A.D., SACKETT, D.L. and GUYATT, G.H. (1993) For the Evidence-Based Medicine Working Group. *Users' Guides to the Medical Literature. I. How to get started.* JAMA 270: 2093–5.
- GUYATT, G.H., SACKETT, D.L. and COOK, D.J. (1993) for the Evidence-Based Medicine Working Group. *Users' Guides to the Medical Literature. II. How to use an article about therapy or prevention: A. Are the results of the study valid?* JAMA 270: 2598–601.
- GUYATT, G.H., SACKETT, D.L. and COOK, D.J. (1994) for the Evidence-Based Medicine Working Group. *Users' Guides to the Medical Literature. II. How to use an article about therapy or prevention: B. What were the results and will they help me in caring for my patients?* JAMA 271: 59–63.
- JAESCHKE, R., GUYATT, G. and SACKETT, D.L. (1994) for the Evidence-Based Medicine Working Group. *Users' Guides to the Medical Literature. III. How to use an article about a diagnostic test: A. Are the results of the study valid?* JAMA 271: 389–91.

- JAESCHKE, R., GUYATT, G.H. and SACKETT, D.L. (1994) for the Evidence-Based Medicine Working Group. *Users' Guides to the Medical Literature. III. How to use an article about a diagnostic test: B. What are the results and will they help me in caring for my patients?* JAMA 271: 703–7.
- LEVINE, M., WALTER, S., LEE, H. et al. (1994) for the Evidence-Based Medicine Working Group. *Users' Guides to the Medical Literature. IV. How to use an article about harm.* JAMA 271: 1615–19.
- LAUPACIS, A., WELLS, G., RICHARDSON, S. and TUGWELL, P. (1994) for the Evidence-Based Medicine Working Group. *Users' Guides to the Medical Literature. V. How to use an article about prognosis.* JAMA 272: 234–7.
- OXMAN, A.D., COOK, D.J. and GUYATT, G.H. (1994) for the Evidence-Based Medicine Working Group. *Users' Guides to the Medical Literature. VI. How to use an overview.* JAMA 272: 1367–71.
- RICHARDSON, W.S. and DETSKY, A.S. (1995) for the Evidence-Based Medicine Working Group. *Users' Guides to the Medical Literature. VII. How to use a clinical decision analysis. A. Are the results of the study valid?* JAMA 273: 1292–5.
- RICHARDSON, W.S. and DETSKY, A.S. (1995) for the Evidence-Based Medicine Working Group. *Users' Guides to the Medical Literature. VII. How to use a clinical decision analysis. B. What are the results and will they help me in caring for my patients?* JAMA 273: 1610–13.
- HAYWARD, R.S., WILSON, M.C., TUNIS, S.R. et al. (1995) for the Evidence-Based Medicine Working Group. *Users' Guides to the Medical Literature. VIII. How to use clinical practice guidelines. A. Are the recommendations valid?* JAMA 274: 570–4.
- WILSON, M.C., HAYWARD, R.S., TUNIS, S.R. et al. (1995) for the Evidence-Based Medicine Working Group. *Users' Guides to the Medical Literature. VIII. How to use clinical practice guidelines. B. What are the recommendations and will they help you in caring for your patients?* JAMA 274: 1630–2.
- GUYATT, G.H., SACKETT, D.L., SINCLAIR, J.C. et al. (1995) for the Evidence-Based Medicine Working Group. *Users' Guides to the Medical Literature. IX. A method for grading health care recommendations.* JAMA 274: 1800–4.
- JAMA (1996) *Erratum: Users' Guides to the Medical Literature. IX. A method for grading health care recommendations: JAMA 274: 1800–4.* JAMA 275: 1232.

- NAYLOR, C.D. and GUYATT, G.H. (1996) for the Evidence-Based Medicine Working Group. *Users' Guides to the Medical Literature. X. How to use an article reporting variations in the outcomes of health services.* JAMA 275: 554–8.
- NAYLOR, C.D. and GUYATT, D.H. (1996) *Users' Guides to the Medical Literature. XI. How to use an article about a clinical utilization review.* JAMA 275: 1435–9.

The *Users' Guides to the Medical Literature* are now available on the World Wide Web, but they are presented in a slightly different format to the paper publications, as follows:

Contents
- Evidence Based Medicine
- Why Users' Guides
- How to get started
- How to use primary studies about:
  - Therapy or prevention
  - Diagnosis
  - Harm
  - Prognosis
- How to use integrative studies that are:
  - Overviews
  - Decision analyses
  - Practice guidelines
  - Utilization analyses
  - Outcome analyses

URL: http://hiru.mcmaster.ca/ebm/userguid/

In fact, the Health Information Resource Unit also provides other high-quality appraisal resources at its Web site: http://hiru.mcmaster.ca

A.2   The Cochrane Library

In The Cochrane Library, the Cochrane Review Methodology Database (CRMD) provides a comprehensive list of articles on the assessment of methodological quality of RCTs (see Appendix I, Section A.1.4).

A.3   Standard texts

The philosophy of science of critical appraisal and its application is best appreciated by reading the classic book on clinical epidemiology:

- SACKETT, D.L., HAYNES, R.B., GUYATT, G.H. and TUGWELL, P. (1991) *Clinical Epidemiology.* Little Brown, Boston, MA.

An excellent review of the skills needed for critical appraisal and evidence-based decision making is provided by:

- EDDY, D.M. (1992) *A Manual for Assessing Health Practices and Designing Practice Policies; the Explicit Approach.* American College of Physicians, Independence Mall West, Sixth Street at Race, Philadelphia, PA 19106-1572, USA.

Eddy discusses topics such as: types of evidence and biases; collecting and interpreting evidence; combining evidence; models for indirect evidence; comparing benefits and harms; costs.

Eddy also tackles the important subject of 'writing, reviewing and disseminating a policy'. This book is strongly recommended.

A.4   *Bandolier*

Bandolier is a monthly newsletter published by the R&D Directorate of the Anglia & Oxford NHS Executive Regional Office. The aim is to provide evidence-based information for purchasers of healthcare and to help develop the searching and appraisal skills of those who make decisions about healthcare and health services (see Box A.III.1).

The title *Bandolier* was chosen because when one of the editors was acting as a purchaser he often felt like the Emperor Maximilian, as painted by Manet, helpless and bound, before a firing squad of providers and professionals armed with bandoliers full of bullets. A typical afternoon for

---

Box A.III.1

The objectives of the editors of *Bandolier* are to support any decision maker in their ability to:

- find the best available evidence on tests and treatments;
- be conversant with the criteria used to appraise trials and systematic reviews on tests and clinical and cost effectiveness;
- define absolute and relative risk and be aware of the strengths and weaknesses of different ways of expressing research results;
- define, calculate and use NNT;
- list screening tests that do more good than harm;
- define odds ratios and know their value;
- define and interpret confidence intervals and power;
- distinguish sensitivity, specificity and predictive value of tests.

a purchaser might be a meeting with orthopaedic surgeons at 2.00 pm, one with cardiologists at 4.00 pm, and lastly one with gastroenterologists, over a sandwich, at 6.30 pm. On each occasion, the provider team is armed with evidence and, frequently, shrouds to wave, whereas the purchaser is rushing from meeting to meeting, topic to topic, often lacking the evidence in a useful form.

Bandolier habitués read it because of its accessible style and the useful information it provides. The editors knew that if they started a newsletter called 'Epidemiologically based techniques for analysing evidence and making evidence-based decisions', it would have gone in the bin in nanoseconds. By addressing topical problems and featuring recently published papers, the editors aim to disseminate the principles of epidemiological techniques without ever using the word 'epidemiology'.

For further details, contact *Bandolier* Editorial Office, Pain Relief Unit, The Churchill Hospital, Oxford, OX3 7LJ; tel. (+44)-1865-226132; fax (+44)-1865-226978; email: andrew.moore%mailgate.jr2@ox.ac.uk; URL: http://www.jr2.ox.ac.uk/Bandolier

B. CRITICAL APPRAISAL SKILLS PROGRAMME – CASP

The Critical Appraisal Skills Programme (CASP) has been running in the Anglia and Oxford Region since 1994. The target audience for CASP are those personnel who must take decisions about groups of patients or populations, rather than individuals. The aim within CASP is to 'help health service decision makers develop skills in the critical appraisal of evidence about effectiveness, in order to promote the delivery of evidence-based healthcare'.

This aim is achieved by means of a cascade of half-day workshops that introduce participants to the key skills necessary to find and make sense of evidence to support decisions about health services. CASP is used to introduce the ideas of evidence-based medicine. As the workshops are focused particularly on the critical appraisal of systematic reviews, CASP is also used to introduce the related ideas of the Cochrane Collaboration (see Appendix I, Box A.I.1).

CASP workshops are promoted by:

- encouraging personnel to identify local training needs in evidence-based healthcare;
- working with local personnel to plan and deliver workshops;
- training local personnel to deliver the workshops;
- working with others to evaluate the delivery and impact of the workshops;
- networking personnel who have been involved in running workshops.

As the primary aim within CASP is to develop skills in critical appraisal, and not to run workshops, cascading the confidence and competence to run workshops is pivotal. The cascade depends on a network of local co-ordinators who convene regular 'training the trainer' sessions for other personnel who are interested in running workshops. Thus far, about 1 in 8 workshop participants have volunteered to help plan and deliver further workshops.

Those making decisions about groups of patients or populations are nearly always generalists who tend to rely on summaries of the evidence rather than on primary research reports. Such summaries may be published under a wide variety of names (e.g. editorials and reviews) and will probably contain evidence about a wide range of issues (e.g. effectiveness, efficiency, equity, appropriateness, acceptability and responsiveness). Whatever the issue, however, appraising the review raises three generic questions.

1. How trustworthy is the review (do I believe it?)?
2. What are the results and how important are they (what does it say?)?
3. What is its relevance to the 'local' situation (how important is it to us?)?

The detailed questions used in CASP workshops to appraise systematic reviews of evidence about effectiveness are shown in Box 5.2.

The approach within CASP is complementary to the work at the Centre for Evidence-Based Medicine in Oxford, and elsewhere, where personnel work directly with clinicians providing healthcare.

The success of CASP in the support of personnel in a wide variety of settings who run critical appraisal workshops illustrates the accessibility and universality of these skills. They are not confined to individuals who have research and/or clinical experience; anyone with common sense and an interest in healthcare can learn how to make sense of evidence and to relate that evidence to the decisions facing them.

For further information about CASP, contact:
Claire Spittlehouse; tel: (+44)-1865-226968;
email: casp@cix.compulink.co.uk;
URL: http://fester.his.path.cam.ac.uk/phealth/casphome/htm

Ruairidh Milne

STORING

As emphasised in the text, it is not possible to store the evidence found in paper form alone. However, it is possible to combine a simple storage system, such as storing paper alphabetically, with the use of a reference or bibliographic management software package.

Reference or bibliographic management software is a specialised database that enables references, once entered, not only to be sorted and edited but also to be produced as bibliographies in the various formats that might be required for different publishers. There is a good background book on reference or bibliographic management software by Terry Hanson.[1]

There are several different types of software: Procite, Papyrus, Idealist, EndNote Plus2 and Reference Manager. Obviously, these change and evolve over time, but it is possible to keep abreast of such developments by reading the UKOLUG Newsletter. This is published bimonthly by the UK Online Users Group (the national user group for online, CD-ROM and Internet searchers). There is an article on bibliographic management software in each issue. By consulting back numbers of the UKOLUG Newsletter it is possible to review the latest version of all the commonly used types of software.

UKOLUG Newsletter is free to members of UKOLUG; it is also possible to subscribe, contact: Christine Baker, The Old Chapel, Walden, West Burton, Leyburn, North Yorkshire, DL8 4LE; tel. & fax: (+44)-1969-663749; email: cabaker@ukolug.demon.co.uk.

The other useful source of advice is the librarian. If you expect to work in one place for a long time, it is often helpful to use the software recommended by the librarian on site; however, as the job market changes and professionals become more 'mobile', it might be best to pick the software that corresponds to your needs and learn how to use it in association with MEDLINE, for example, so that you can carry your own library with you.

Reference

1. HANSON, T. (Editor) (1995) *Bibliographic Software and the Electronic Library.* University of Herefordshire Press, Hatfield.

IMPLEMENTING

In the UK, the basic functions of the National R&D Programme include:

- the promotion of an evidence-based culture;
- the promotion of the implementation of research findings.

Driven by the R&D Programme, under the leadership of Sir Michael Peckham, other sectors of the NHS are responding to this challenge such that the implementation of research findings and evidence-based decision making are now much higher on the agenda than they were hitherto.

Since 1990, several approaches towards the implementation of research findings have been developed, and there are now examples of ways in which evidence-based decision making is being used towards this end. It is possible to characterise these different approaches as follows:

- proactive;
- reactive;
- opportunistic;
- the use of 'managed' care as a framework.

A. PROACTIVE APPROACHES

Within a proactive approach, new knowledge derived from research is promoted vigorously to ensure that it is incorporated into clinical practice more quickly than would have occurred by the haphazard and slow process of diffusion. Although this type of approach was piloted and has been studied most in Canada,[1] it has recently been developed in the UK within such projects as the GRiPP Project (see Section A.1) and a project known as the PACE Programme (see Section A.2).

A.1   Main lessons learnt from the GRiPP Project

The GRiPP Project is described in Section 7.3.5.

A.1.1   Choosing the topic

- Be explicit about the criteria and ensure it is possible to defend them.
- Consider how the main stakeholders will react to the choice.
- Involve those stakeholders in the choice right from the beginning.
- Do not rush into a choice; ensure *all* the criteria have been considered.

A.1.2   Consulting and involving local professionals

- Ensure *all* the key players, both clinical and managerial, are involved.
- Involve all key players early on in the process.
- Ensure that communication with the professions and the managers is undertaken frequently from the beginning of the process.
- Communications should include the choice of topic (what and why), the nature of the evidence, and the (draft) outputs of the project.
- Ensure channels of communication do not become crossed or confused.
- Not everyone who is involved needs to be an active participant of the project group; keep the group small enough for it to be productive.

A.1.3   Reviewing the evidence

- Maintain a balance between the strength of the evidence base and the efforts that are put into other elements of the GRiPP process.
- Do not expect this process to yield the precise answers that clinicians and purchasers might at first anticipate from the evidence.
- Involve clinicians in the whole process of evidence review in order to enhance the validity, credibility, and acceptance of the project.
- Consider whether the evidence available locally needs to be reviewed, and if so who should do it, to what extent, and why (e.g. to enhance local expertise).
- When using a locally produced evidence base, ensure it undergoes adequate peer review.

A.1.4   Acquiring baseline data

- Decide at an early stage why data are to be collected (e.g. to help choose the topic, to compare current with ideal practice, to establish a baseline and monitor later improvements, to raise awareness among clinicians).
- Plan (with the involvement of clinicians) how and when data will be collected, both before and after the project.
- Do not embark on a large data-gathering exercise without rigorous review of the aims, objectives and methods.
- Do not let data gathering become an end in itself.
- The skills of local audit facilitators can be very helpful in a GRiPP project.

A.1.5   Developing evidence-based guidelines

- Those responsible for producing guidelines should put into practice the well-established evidence about the factors determining success in the development and implementation of guidelines; see, for example, *Implementing Clinical Practice Guidelines*, Effective Health Care Bulletin Number 8, York, 1994.
- Do not expect to implement 'imported' guidelines; they will usually need to be adapted, not merely adopted. Guidelines may, however, be based on evidence authoritatively reviewed elsewhere.
- Most guidelines will be more effective if their development involves all the relevant disciplines engaged in the care of that group of patients, including 'front line' staff who will have to use the guidelines and relevant managers.
- If sufficient care is taken with the other elements of the process (e.g. choosing a topic that the clinicians believe to be important, gaining acceptance of the research evidence, linking the guidelines to established audit groups), then the guidelines are more likely to be used.
- Establish and monitor a system to ensure that the guidelines are based on the best evidence available, and are not a justification *post hoc* of current practice.
- Ensure that the guidelines are not biased in favour of well-researched, as opposed to clinically important, areas of practice; this will require a system for grading both clinical importance and the strength of evidence.

A.1.6   Disseminating and implementing

- Plan a dissemination strategy from the beginning of the project, and review it continuously.
- Much effort (and resource) is necessary to present the research findings in a 'user friendly' way to suit the varying needs of different audiences who will be expected to accept and implement the findings within a variety of contexts.
- To be credible and gain acceptance, the product needs to be appropriate in terms of the message (e.g. authoritative, realistic) and the format (e.g. neither too glossy nor too shabby).
- Consider disseminating information to patients early on in the process.
- Utilise the communication channels and change management strategies that already exist: the use of the audit network to implement GRiPP among clinicians is a good example; the involvement of clinical directors in the commissioning process may be another.
- Explore the links between the results of the project and the process of healthcare commissioning, i.e. between the clinical and contractual implications. Assume that those links are problematic, and act accordingly until proven otherwise.

A.1.7   Evaluation

- It is important to evaluate such projects, and to plan the evaluation from the beginning as an integral part of the project.
- The evaluation should take note of:
  - the scientific rigour of the evidence and guidelines (e.g. the need for peer review);
  - the outcome in terms of clinical behaviour and health status;
  - the organisational and political effects of the project, including all the elements of the project.

  It should have both quantitative and qualitative elements and be formative not summative (i.e. should be designed to help the project develop rather than to act as a final judgement on its success).
- Such evaluation of local projects need not be elaborate but based on relatively simple systematic checks on progress.

- The main participants should be involved in the evaluation.
- More formal, summative evaluation of the impact of projects such as GRiPP is needed, and should be funded centrally so that it can be designed with adequate controls and comparisons across a variety of sites.

A.1.8   Project management

- Do everything possible to ensure that all the key stakeholders are involved and are kept informed of the process throughout.
- Treat the project as a change management exercise, requiring, for example:
  - a committed and influential change management team;
  - time and resources to secure the changes;
  - a clear and shared vision of what the change is trying to achieve;
  - a thorough analysis of the current situation including the attitudes and interests of all the key actors;
  - a well-planned and closely managed overall strategy;
  - clear and closely monitored intermediate steps for achieving that strategy;
  - excellent communication among *all* those involved in the change.

Sections A.1.1–A.1.8 have been adapted from a report entitled 'Learning from the GRiPP Project — an executive summary' by John Gabbay and Sue Dopson which was written for Oxford Regional Health Authority.

A.2   The PACE Programme

The PACE Programme (Promoting Action on Clinical Effectiveness) is part of a new medical development initiative by the King's Fund. The PACE Programme builds on the GRiPP project (Oxford) and the FACTS project (Sheffield), and has been designed to complement the work within the NHS Research and Development Strategy to understand the issues involved in implementing research findings. The aim is to generate a network of projects to demonstrate the effective implementation of evidence-based practice and identify the factors for success.

The programme has three main elements:

- a series of local projects to explore the issues involved in using research-based information about clinical effectiveness to improve services to patients;
- networks of people who are interested in the promotion of evidence-based practice to support the sharing of the lessons and experiences from the local work;
- a series of publications to disseminate the lessons learned to those in the NHS concerned with evidence-based healthcare.

The programme includes 16 projects — two in each NHS region. The projects will run for 2 years in order to include preparatory work as well as monitoring the impact on local services and the evaluation of results.

The planning guidelines of the NHS now encourage each health authority to negotiate with service providers specific targets for either increasing or decreasing certain types of intervention for their population. In EL(94)74, the NHS Executive emphasised the UK Government's commitment to improving the effectiveness of clinical services and listed sources of clinical effectiveness information.

A PACE Bulletin is produced quarterly and circulated to chief executives of health authorities and NHS Trusts. Copies are also sent to individual personnel interested in the network. Address: King's Fund Development Centre, 11–13 Cavendish Square, London W1M 0AN; tel: (+44)-171-307-2694; fax: (+44)-171-307-2810. URL: http://libsun1.jr2.ox.ac.uk/nhserdd/aordd/evidence/PACE.HTM

B. THE REACTIVE APPROACH

Those who make decisions about healthcare services for groups of patients or populations must be prepared to make proactive decisions on the basis of evidence. However, it is possible that by the time a new proposal has been brought to the attention of purchasers, it may already have been offered to the population; in this situation it may be difficult to stop providing the service. It is paramount that such interventions should be withdrawn or their use actively and increasingly restricted. Such 'remedial' action must be undertaken as soon as possible after uncontrolled introduction.

An essential pre-requisite for those who are concerned to promote evidence-based healthcare is foresight such that they are able to envisage and predict potential future developments. For example, two neonatal screening tests are currently being offered routinely: for hypothyroidism and for phenylketonuria; however, some biochemists are experimenting with screening tests for eight other metabolic diseases and this information is freely available on the clinical biochemists' mailbase. If purchasers in public health are to take pre-emptive action and manage the introduction of these new tests, or even prevent them from being introduced, it is important to be aware of such developments and the way in which they might unfold.

C. OPPORTUNISTIC IMPLEMENTATION

Both proactive and reactive evidence-based decision making have as a focus specific innovations, either innovations of knowledge in a proactive approach or the introduction of innovations in technology in a reactive approach. Although both these approaches are important ways of implementing research evidence, it is also important to be able to exploit opportunities as they arise and to identify ways in which decisions that would otherwise be dominated by resource constraints or values can be transformed into those based on evidence.

Almost all health services worldwide are subject to financial pressure. This has led to the prioritisation of healthcare delivery, and in some countries to explicit rationing of both primary and secondary care.[1, 2] Much of the debate about prioritisation and rationing is concerned with the ethical aspects of decision making, but it is important to recognise the opportunities for promoting evidence-based decision making when these debates are taking place.

In the past, such debates were not as common; when they did occur, the resolution was often a matter of identifying interventions that had no beneficial effect and either preventing their introduction or promoting their cessation. Nowadays, however, the agenda is different: a situation may arise in which there are no interventions for which evidence of effectiveness is completely lacking, but some of the evidence may be of low quality, such as that derived from a series of cases as opposed to that derived from a systematic review of RCTs. Moreover, if clinicians have gained experience from a series of cases, an attempt to stop the provision of a service or to adjust the rate of provision of that service to a national rate may be resisted because the clinicians are convinced patients will benefit from their care. Thus, it is often necessary not simply to identify ineffective interventions but to assess a wide range of interventions by determining the magnitude of the beneficial effect and that of the adverse effect and weighing the balance of benefit to harm against the cost of achieving the benefit.

In future, the greatest opportunities for evidence-based decision making may arise as financial pressures increase. Although these decisions can be dominated by economists or ethicists, the health service decision maker who knows how to find, appraise and apply evidence to the care of populations will find an influential, if not always comfortable, place at the decision-making table.

References

1. CRISP, R., HOPE, T. and GIBBS, D. (1996) *The Asbury draft policy on the ethical use of resources.* Br. Med. J. 312: 1528–31.
2. NEW, B. (1996) on behalf of the Rationing Agenda Group. *The rationing agenda in the NHS.* Br. Med. J. 312: 1593–601.

D. THE RISE OF 'MANAGED CARE'

Opportunities for implementing research-based evidence are also offered by the trend towards 'managed care' in which a systematic approach to care management is taken and greater use is made of clinical guidelines.

At present, this trend is most marked in the USA[1] where there is now a wide range of different approaches to regulating care. Two different strategies have emerged:

1. to ensure that doctors are not paid in such a way as to distort their decision making;
2. to use the opportunities offered by managed care to promote evidence-based decision making.

However, one of the fears of the medical profession is that evidence-based healthcare will be used as a means of removing individual professional liberty. This debate is most lively in the USA in response to the greater control exerted there, but it is also beginning to be joined in other countries as different techniques, such as the production of 'critical pathways', are introduced by those who manage or purchase healthcare.[2] In the UK, the development of clinical guidelines is being pursued in the independent healthcare sector.[3]

Although these opportunities to influence the delivery of healthcare are tempting, their realisation must be tempered with the knowledge that most clinical decisions cannot be governed by strict rules; guidelines have to remain as guidelines. The introduction of managed care is undoubtedly changing the role of the physician[4] and although change is necessary it is vital that one of the most important, but under-valued and under-evaluated, aspects of medical care — the bond between clinician and patient — is not disrupted.

References

1. SWARTZ, K. and BRENNAN, T.A. (1996) *Integrated health care, capitated payment, and quality: the role of regulation.* Ann. Intern. Med. 124: 442–8.
2. PEARSON, S.D., GOULART-FISHER, D. and LEE, T.H. (1995) *Critical pathways as a strategy for improving care: problems and potential.* Ann. Intern. Med. 123: 941–9.
3. FAIRFIELD, G. and WILLIAMS, R. (1996) *Clinical guidelines in the independent health care sector [Editorial].* Br. Med. J. 312: 1554–5.
4. SELKER, H.P. (1996) *Capitated payment for medical care and the role of the physician [Editorial].* Ann. Intern. Med. 124: 449–51.

Further reading

APPLEBY, J., WALSHE, K. and HAM, C. (1995) *Acting on the evidence. A review of clinical effectiveness: sources of information, dissemination and implementation.* Research Paper Number 17, National Association of Health Authorities and Trusts (NAHAT), Birmingham.

Page numbers in *italics* refer to boxes and tables, and those in **bold** type to figures.

absolute risk *see* risk
abstracts, misleading 63–4
abstracts *see also ACP Journal Club*; DARE
abuse, and gastrointestinal illness, review of 72
acceptability
   in appraisal of new treatments *163*
   in evidence on quality *144*
   sources of information on 226
access to services, patient expectations for 6
ACP Journal Club
   abstracts in 232
   advice on searching for evidence 30, 42
   and DARE 224
adaptive design, and significant effect of treatment 79
adverse effects of interventions
   and effectiveness 116
   and patient choice 204
   and safety 122
   studies on 87–8, 89, 124
adverse effects of interventions *see also* outcome; safety;
      side-effects
age, and heart failure, applicability of results on 109
age *see also* elderly people
air pollutants, MEDLINE search strategy for
      information on 236–7
alcohol misuse
   and *Effective Health Care* bulletins 226
   healthcare needs assessment 229
American College of Physicians (ACP) Journal Club
      see ACP Journal Club
anaesthesia, prospective studies in, in research on
      safety 124
analysis techniques, and systematic reviews 73
angina, and necessity for exercise stress tests 151
Anglia & Oxford NHS Executive Regional Office
   and *Bandolier* 242
   and CASP 243–5
   and development of evidence-based healthcare xv
anthropological studies, and healthcare policy 56
antibiotic resistance, and clinical practice 24
antihypertensive agents, and myocardial infarction
      87–8
anxiety, and patient choice 210–12
aortic aneurism, doubtfulness of screening for *178*

applicability of evidence 83, 109–10, 110–11, 197
   on appropriateness 152
   on cost-effectiveness 138–9
   on effectiveness 113, 119, 125
   and patient choice 110–11, 207
   on patient satisfaction 130–1
   on policy making 187–8
   on quality of care 145–7
   on safety 125
appraisal
   of service options, assessment reviews on 229
   of systematic reviews 74–7
   training in 66
appraisal of evidence xi-xii, 68, 239–45
appraisal of evidence
   on appropriateness 151–2
   by purchasers *242*
   on cost-effectiveness 138
   on effectiveness of interventions 116–17, 176
   for evidence-based primary care 169, *170*
   in management skills 2–3, 56, 157, 161, 196–8
   and patient choice 204
   on patient satisfaction 130
   on policy making 2–3, 56, 96–8, 161, 187
   on qualitative research 101
   on quality of research 69–101
   on quality standards 144–5
   on risk in public health policies 190
   on safety 123–4
   on screening 49–51
   on study type 81–2, *83*, 88–9, 91–2
   on tests 43–4, *45*
   on therapy 30–3
appropriateness
   appraisal of evidence on 151–2, *152*
   dimensions of 147–51
asking questions, in evidence-based decision-making 2
aspirin, after myocardial infarction, public education
      concerning 24
Association for Health Services Research, USA 234
asthma
   MEDLINE search strategy for information on 236–7
   in Priority Research Programmes *227*
audit
   of clinical decision-making 166, 202
   evidence-based 159–61
   for reduction of unproven interventions 24, 27
   in searching for evidence on quality standards 144, 145

back pain
  reviews of variations in 228
  and treatment after diagnostic tests 39–40, 42
backache, and epidural anaesthesia, prospective studies
      on 124
balance of good and harm see good:harm balance
Bandolier newsletter
  and development of appraisal skills 169, 170
  and evidence-based information for purchasers
      242–3
barriers
  to clinical practice 214, 215
  to management skills 195
benefit
  and appropriateness 148
  and effectiveness 117
  and necessity 150
  and patient choice 204
bias
  in abstracts 63–4
  as barrier to good clinical practice 215
  in evidence on effectiveness 116, 117, 117
  and funding of research 133–4
  in outcome of new treatments 104
  in publication of research 61
  in systematic reviews 72–3
  in trial results 78, 81, 88–9, 223
bias see also patient selection
bibliographic management software 247
blood pressure, screening tests 37–8, 47
BMJ see British Medical Journal
breast biopsy, after diagnostic tests 42
breast cancer
  patient choice in treatment 212
  screening 47, 48
    Breast Screening Programme 140, 141
    doubtfulness of benefits of 178
    framing effect on results of 85
    and patient demands 6
breast implants, and autoimmune disease, litigation
      concerning 193
British Medical Association (BMA) library, on
      evidence-based primary care 169
British Medical Journal (BMJ), searching for information
      in 62, 63
British Medical Journal (BMJ) Publishing Group 222
budgetary pressures see finance; resources

CABG (coronary artery bypass grafting) 143, 146–7, 228
Caesarian sections, and purchasers' requirements 175
cancer
  apparent epidemics of and public health 189
  assessment of appropriateness of treatment 147–8
  disclosure of and patient choice 211–12
cancer see also individual types
cardiac interventions, benefit of 118
cardiac rehabilitation, framing effect on results of 85
cardiac surgery, after diagnostic tests 42
cardiopulmonary resuscitation (CPR), and patient
      choice 206

cardiovascular disease
  effect of cholesterol-lowering treatments 106
  mega trials on management of 79
  in Priority Research Programmes 227
cardiovascular disease see also individual conditions
      & coronary heart disease
carotid artery stenosis, applicability of research
      findings 110–11
case-control studies
  dimensions of 87–8
  evidence on 88–9
  in observational research 71
  in research on effectiveness 116
  in research on safety 123
  for risk factors in public health 188, 189
  in studies of health service organisation 32
  term from MEDLINE 231
  uses and abuses of 89
CASP, critical appraisal skills programme 243–45
cataract
  management of
    and Effective Health Care bulletins 226
    and healthcare needs assessment 229
CCTR (Cochrane Controlled Trials Register) 222, 225
CD-ROM users group 247
CDSR see Cochrane Database of Systematic Reviews
central policy, in Priority Research Programmes 227
Centre for Evidence-Based Medicine 244
cervical screening
  incentive payments for 217
  outcome measures in 48, 140
chemotherapy, assessment of appropriateness of
      147–8
chest pain
  clinical innovations in management of 165
  patient expectations in treatment of 4
  volume of treatment after tests 41
chief executives, management skills of 3, 156–7
child health
  healthcare needs assessment 229
  information and guidance on 225
  in Priority Research Programmes 227
childbirth
  maternal care in, reviews of variations in 228
  value of emotional support during 115
childhood leukaemia, reviews of variations in 228
children, unintentional injuries to, and Effective Health
      Care bulletins 226
chlamydia in pregnancy, unproven value of screening
      for 23, 176
cholesterol screening
  and Effective Health Care bulletins 226
  whole population, unproven value of 23, 176
Churchill Livingstone
  publishers of Effective Health Care 226
  publishers of evidence-based healthcare journals
      232
  publishers of Evidence-Based Medicine:
      How to Practice and Teach EBM 235
cigarette advertising, and values in policy making 192
clinical audit, need for evidence in 159–60, 161

clinical decision-making
   failures in 214
   and healthcare policy 201
   types of 202–3
clinical development directorate, roles of 166
Clinical Effectiveness Initiative 182–3
Clinical Epidemiology, on critical appraisal 241
clinical innovations, in evidence-based needs
      assessment 172, 174–7
clinical outcome *see* outcome
clinical policies, development of 217–18, **219**
clinical practice
   evidence-based 213–15
   evolution of 24–5, 163–4, 165–6, 216–19
   impact of on healthcare costs 25–7
clinical practice guidelines, and *Effective Health Care*
      bulletins 226
Clinical Standards Advisory Group reports 228
clinical trials
   promotion of 25, 177, 177–8, *178*
   systematic review of, computer access to 59
   terms from MEDLINE *231*
clinical trials *see also* research
clinician's conundrum, on applicability of findings
      110–111
clotbusting agents *see* thrombolysis
co-morbidity, and outcome 143
Cochrane, A., on efficiency 135
Cochrane Centres *223*
Cochrane Collaboration 61, 62, 222–3
   on effectiveness of training for evidence-based
         decision-making 161, *162*
   in search for evidence on RCTs 80
   on search strategies 235–7
   on search for systematic reviews 74, 77
Cochrane Collaboration Handbook 223, 235–7
Cochrane Controlled Trials Register (CCTR) 222, 225
Cochrane Database of Systematic Reviews (CDSR) 61,
      74, 222–3
   in the evidence centre 158
   for evidence on effectiveness 115
Cochrane Database of Systematic Reviews Handbook 117
Cochrane Library *8*, 77
   for evidence on RCTs 81
   for evidence on systematic reviews 59, 221, 222–3
   of information for evidence-based primary care 169
   on search strategies 235–7
Cochrane Review Methodology Database (CRMD) 222,
      225, 241
coeliac disease, MEDLINE search for a test for *42*
cognitive therapy, in MUPS 14–15
cohort studies 71, 89–92
   for effectiveness 116
   on health service organisation 32
   for risk factors in public health 188, 189
   for safety 31, 123
   shortcomings of in appraisal of evidence on
         screening 49
   and surveys 94
   term from MEDLINE *231*
   uses and abuses of 92

Collaborative Review Groups *223*
colorectal cancer
   healthcare needs assessment 229
   unproven value of screening for 23, *176*, *178*
commissioning, evidence-based decisions in 171–82
communication
   in clinical decision-making 127, 202, 203
   in implementation of evidence 250, 252
   and patient choice 207, **208–9**, 210
   and patient satisfaction 127
community health care, evidence-based primary care in
      167–70
compensation or failure, patient expectations for 6
competence
   in clinical practice 214
   in management skills 7, 195–6, 197
competencies, in reference management systems 198–9
'compleat healthcare manager' 199
computer systems
   and access to evidence 59, 159
   requirements of for the Cochrane Library 222
   storage systems *8*, 198–9, 247–8
   use of in primary care 170
confidence intervals, in applicability of research results
      76, 104–8, 119
congenital biliary atresia, unproven value of screening
      for 23, *176*
consumerism, and patient expectations in healthcare
      6, 18
controlled trials
   bibliography of 225
   in research on effectiveness 116
coronary angiography, increase in after tests 41
coronary artery bypass grafting (CABG)
   and mortality rates 143, 146–7
   reviews of variations in 228
coronary artery disease programme, cost-benefit study
      of 138–9
coronary heart disease, healthcare needs assessment 229
coronary heart disease *see also* cardiovascular disease
corticosteroids in preterm labour, effectiveness of *178*
cost
   advantage of case-control studies 88
   in clinical decisions 201
   in healthcare policy xiii-xiv 3, 12, 17–18, 20, 54, 229
   impact of technological developments on healthcare
      5–6
   influences on 25–7
   in medical education 217
   in new treatments, appraisal of 148, *163*
   in screening, appraisal of 39, *51*, 96, *98*
cost *see also* finance
cost-benefit analysis, in economic evaluations 137
cost-effectiveness 133–7
   analysis, in economic evaluations 137
   applicability of evidence on 138–9
   and managed care plan *180*
   Register of Cost-Effectiveness Studies 232
   and risk in public health policies 190
   searching for evidence on 138, 226
cost-effectiveness *see also* economic appraisal

cost-utility analysis 112
counselling services, patient expectations for 6
coverage criteria, in insurance-based funding 179–8
CRD *see* NHS Centre for Reviews and Dissemination
(NHS CRD)
critical appraisal, reading list for 239–43
critical appraisal skills programme (CASP) 243–5
CRMD (Cochrane Review Methodology Database)
222, 225, 241
cultural effects, of RCTs 83–4
culture, in an evidence-based organisation 156
cystic fibrosis, reviews of variations in 228

DARE (Database of Abstracts of Reviews of
Effectiveness) 74, 115, 222, 224
database of current health services research (HSRProj),
in USA 234
databases
in search for systematic reviews 72, 74
subject specialist 230–2
databases *see also* CDSR; DARE; EMBASE; MEDLINE
decision analysis 94–6
appraisal of evidence on 96–8
uses and abuses of 99
decision tree, construction of 94–5
decision-making xi-xii, xviii, 1–3, 199
barriers to 7–8
'black belt' decision-making **181**, 182
and CASP programmes 243–5
ethics in 255
in managed care 256–7
opportunistic 255–6
and politics 28
pro-active 249–54
reactive 254–5
training for 161, *162*
deep vein thrombosis
and oral contraceptives, cohort studies on 123
risk of treatment and patient choice 207
degree of surprise, in analysis of disease clusters 189
dementia, healthcare needs assessment 229
dental anaesthesia, reviews of variations in 228
dentistry, in care of older people 5
dentists' trial, of interpersonal relationships of care
115, 131
depression, and *Effective Health Care* bulletins 226
descriptive studies, in evidence on healthcare
policy 55
Development and Education Committee of Wessex
Regional Health Authority 227
diabetes
healthcare needs assessment 229
variations in management of 228
diagnosis, MeSH headings for 43
diagnostic tests *see* tests
dilatation and curettage
effectiveness of *178*
and purchasers' requirements 175
disability
as outcome *146*
in Priority Research Programmes *227*

disease
causation of, and case-control studies 87, 88
clusters, statistical analysis of 189–90
management systems 13–15, 172–4
outcomes of 103
dissemination strategy, in implementation of
evidence 252
disutilities, in decision analysis 95, 96, *98*
'doing the right things' 3, 18–20
'doing the right things right' 16, 17–27
'doing things right' 3, 18
Donabedian, Avedis, on healthcare evaluation 139,
140–1, 148
double blind trials 78
Down's syndrome screening
decision tree in 95–6, **97**
doubtfulness of value of *178*
drug abuse, healthcare needs assessment 229
drugs
need for evidence-based decision making about 162–4
purchasing of, and cost control 201
trials of, in RCTs 78, 80

economic appraisal
checklist for *138*
and QALY 112
in research 71, 137
in systematic reviews 74
economic appraisal *see also* cost-effectiveness
economic constraints, and changes in clinical
practice 216
Economics and Operational Research Division
of the Department of Health 232
editorials, shortcomings of *223*
education
clinicians' needs xii, 24, **202**, 216
public needs 24
resources for, and the clinical development
directorate 166
in searching skills 66
Effective Health Care, CRD publication 226
effectiveness 113–14
appraisal of evidence on 116–17
in decision-making 254–6
evidence for, in audit 159
and healthcare policy xiv
observational studies of 118–19
promotion of in the NHS 182–3
reviews of variations in 228
of screening 47, 176
searching for evidence on 115
sources of information on 224, 225–6
of treatment *see* outcome
Effectiveness Matters, CRD publication 225–6
efficacy, and effectiveness 113
efficiency
and cost-effectiveness 134–5
and effectiveness 113
evaluation of 137
and healthcare policy 17–18, 54

elderly people
  dentistry for 5
  falls by 160, *161*, 226
  in Priority Research Programmes *227*
electronic databases, limitations of 62, 62–3
electronic information sources 61, 62
electronic updates, on evidence-based healthcare xvii
EMBASE (Elsevier Science's bibliographic database) 230
  on effectiveness 115
  for evidence-based primary care 168
  on patient satisfaction 129
  in resources for decision makers *8*, 196
  for reviews 74, 221
  shortcomings of *223*
emotional support *see* interpersonal relationships of care
environmental pollutants, MEDLINE search strategy
        for information on 236–7
environmental protection, as public health
        interventions 188
epidemiology, in healthcare decision-making 3, 188–90,
        228–9
epidural anaesthesia, and backache, prospective studies
        on 124
equity, definition of 112
error, in trials 78
ethics
  in clinical trials 69, *70*
  in decision-making 255
ethnicity and health, information and guidance on 225
evaluation, of projects in implementation of evidence
        252–3
evidence
  access to 9, 158–9
  appraisal of xi–xii, 2, 68, 239–45, 250
  difficulty in retrieval of, as barrier to good clinical
        practice *215*
  implementation of 9, 159–61, 249–57
  and legislation in promotion of public health 191
  production of, in evidence-based healthcare 8–9
  retrieval *see also* searching
  searching for xi–xii, 59–66, 235–7
  sources of 221–34
  storage of 198–9, 247–8
    for decision makers *8*, 158
    for training for evidence-based decision-making 161
  strength of *61*
  on tests, searching for and appraisal of 42–4
  unpublished 61–2, 74, *75*, 77, 233–4
  use of evidence, training for evidence-based
        decision-making 161
evidence *see also* information
evidence centre, components of 158–9
evidence management skills 194–9
evidence-based clinical audit 159–61
evidence-based clinical practice 3, 9, 213–15
evidence-based decision making
  by the chief executive 156–7
  in management change 66
  need for xi–xiv, 1–3
  and skills needed for critical appraisal 242
  on therapy 29–33
  training for 161, *162*

evidence-based guidelines, implementation of 169,
        170, 251
evidence-based health service, components of 155–67
evidence-based healthcare 3, 8–15
  in managed care 11–12
  for management of fractured femur 160, *161*
  and patient choice 203–12
  in primary care 167–70
Evidence-Based Healthcare Toolbox, on the
        World Wide Web xvii
evidence-based insurance 179–81
evidence-based litigation 192–3
Evidence-Based Medicine: How to Practice and Teach EBM
        xvii, 235
Evidence-Based Medicine, journal of 232
Evidence-Based Medicine Working Group, guides to
        medical literature 239–41
evidence-based organisations
  components of 154–8
  systems for 158–67
evidence-based policy making 9–12, 183–92
evidence-based process measures 141
evidence-based purchasing 171–82
Excerpta Medica database 230
exercise stress tests, necessity for in angina 151
experience, and clinical decision-making **202**
experimental research *see* research
experimental studies, on effectiveness 117–18
expert committees, reports of, in evidence on
        effectiveness 116
expert opinion, in legal cases 192–3

FACTS project 253
falls in the elderly 160, *161*, 226
false-negative test results 35–6, 39
false-positive test results 35–6, **38**, 39, 40–1
familial hypercholesterolaemia, case-finding for 47
family planning, healthcare needs assessment 229
Filofax, uses of *65*, 66, 170
finance, in decision-making in healthcare 183, 184–8,
        255–6
finance *see also* cost; resources
finance directors, management skills of 3
financing, of the health service 10, 54, 91, 179–81
finding evidence, and use of this book xi–xii
fractured femur, evidence-based criteria for
        management of 160, *161*
fragile X, doubtfulness of screening for *178*
framing effect, bias produces by 84–6, 117
friendly dentists' trial 115, 131
funding, of the health service 10, 54, 91, 179–81

gaps, in requirements for research-based
        knowledge 60–1
gastric surgery, after diagnostic tests *42*
gastrointestinal illness, and abuse, review of 72
general practice, evidence-based primary care in
        167–70
general practitioner, fundholding by 10, 185–7

genetics, and health 13
getting research into purchasing and practice (GRiPP) 178–9, 249–53
glue ear, management of *178*, 226
good:harm balance 20–5, 31
  in appropriateness 147–50
  in clinical decision-making 214
  in clinical innovations 174, 176
  and managed care plan *180*
  in outcomes 103–4, 108–9
  in screening programmes 48–9
good, concept of in healthcare 19
good *see also* good:harm balance
GP *see* general practitioner
GRiPP (getting research into purchasing and practice) 178–9, 249–53
grommets for glue ear, effectiveness of *178*
guidelines
  in implementation of evidence 251
  influence on healthcare policy 218
Guidelines for Meta-analyses Evaluating Diagnostic Tests 43, *44*

hand searching
  in Cochrane Collaboration 77
  for evidence on RCTs 80–1
harm
  concept of in healthcare 19
  as effect of therapy 31
  as side-effect of screening 48–9, *51*, *53*
harm *see also* adverse effects; good:harm ratio; side-effects
HealthSTAR, database on healthcare planning and facilities *8*, 56, 230
health authorities, in health service purchasing 10
Health Technology Assessment Programme, on promoting trials 177
healthcare xiii–xiv, 13
  needs and demands for 4–7, 228–9
  outcome of 12, 20–5
  prioritisation of 255–6
healthcare management
  cohort studies on 90–1, 92
  cost control in 25–7
  innovations in 31–3
  purchasing decisions in xiii–xiv, xviii
  and qualitative research 99–101
  skills of individuals 194–9
  and surveys 93–4
  to increase good:harm ratio 20–5
  and training for evidence-based decision-making 161, *162*
healthcare organisations, need for critical appraisal skills in 198
healthcare policy xi–xii, 55
  changes in 55–6, 57, 112
  and clinical decisions 201
  decision-making in 54–57, 242
  dimensions of appraisal, of tests 43–4
healthcare services 196, 229

economic factors in 137, 217–18
  and promotion of trials 25
  requirements for research-based knowledge 59–61
  variations in outcome in 145
heart failure
  allocation of resources for treatment of 173
  applicability of results on 109
hernia repair, healthcare needs assessment 229
high blood pressure, lack of awareness of evidence on treatment of 204, **205**
hip joint prosthesis, healthcare needs assessment *70*, 229
HSRProj (database of current health services research), USA 234
human frailty, and searching for information 64
human papilloma virus, unproven value of routine screening for *23*, *176*, *178*
hypertension, benefit of preventive interventions 117
hypochondriasis 14
hypothesis-testing research 69–70

illness, in healthcare 13–15
immunisation programmes 137, 188
implementation of evidence 249–57
  about therapy 33
  of effectiveness in the NHS 182–3
  in healthcare changes 199
  opportunistically 255–6
  of research findings 249–57
Implementing Clinical Practice Guidelines 251
impotence, risk of from thiazide 122
inborn errors of metabolism, neonatal screening for *178*
incentives, in clinical practice 216–19
indexing
  inadequate
    as barrier to good clinical practice *215*
    and difficulty in searching for evidence 30, 62, 64, 80
inflation, and healthcare costs 25, **26**, 201
information
  access to, and evidence-based primary care 168–70
  and patient satisfaction 126–7
  retrieval
    and the librarian 65
    problems in 59–64
    and searching skills 65–6
  retrieval *see also* searching
  storage of 66, 247–8
    for evidence-based primary care 169, 170
information *see also* evidence
innovations *see* clinical innovations
inputs, and efficiency in healthcare 18
insulinoma, clinical innovations in diagnosis of *165*
insurance companies
  in health service purchasing xiv, 10, 179–81
  influence on healthcare by 218
intensive care admissions, and research trials *70*, 90
intention to treat, randomisation 78
international trials, problems of 79

Internet
  and information for evidence-based primary care
    168, 169
  users group 247
interobserver variability
  in clinical decision-making 202
  in interpretation of perceptual tests 38–9
interpersonal relationships of care, and patient
    satisfaction 115, 127, 128, 129, 131–2
interpretation
  of information, and patient choice 207
  of RCTs 83–4
interventions, ineffective, elimination of 13
interviews, in qualitative research 100
intraobserver variability, in clinical decision-making 202
Journal of Evidence-Based Healthcare Policy 232

journals
  and changes in clinical practice 165
  in the evidence centre 158
  and evidence from primary research 221
  scanning in searching for evidence by managers 196
  and searching for information 62
  of secondary publication 232

knee replacement, healthcare needs assessment 229
knowledge
  and changes in clinical practice 165–6
  and effectiveness in the NHS 182–3
  as purpose of research 69
knowledge management 65–6

Lancet, searching for information in 62, *63*
laparoscopic cholecystectomy
  evaluation of 24
  patient choice about 206, *207*
lawyers, influence of on patient satisfaction 128
lawyers *see also* legal system; litigation
lead-time bias, in appraisal of evidence on screening
    49–50
leaflets, and patient choice 207, **208–9**
league tables 142–4, 145
  and appropriateness in health care 149
  statistical approaches to analysis of 190
learning difficulties, healthcare needs assessment 229
learning disability services, evidence-based primary
    care in 167–70
legal cases, expert opinion in 192–3
legal system, and interobserver variability 39
legal system *see also* lawyers; litigation
legislation, in promotion of public health 191–2
leukaemia, childhood, reviews of variations in 228
librarian
  as information broker 65
  in resources
    for decision makers *8*
    for evidence on RCTs 80
    for managers 195, 196

on software for storage of information 247
  in training in searching skills 66
library
  and access to information on evidence 9
  as an evidence centre 159
  and the clinical development directorate 166
  and evidence-based primary care 168, 169, 170
  inaccessible, as barrier to good clinical practice *215*
life expectancy in information, and patient choice
    204, 206
lifestyle habits, and health xiii, 13
litigation
  evidence-based 192–3
  fear of and clinical decision-making 7, **202**, 211
  likelihood of 50
litigation *see also* lawyers; legal system
local factors
  in appraisal of evidence *75, 77*, 119, 197
  in CASP programmes 244
  in cost-effectiveness 138–9
  in evidence-based decision-making 2
  in implementation of evidence 33, 250
local factors *see also* applicability
lung cancer, healthcare needs assessment 229

McMaster University, and development of
    evidence-based healthcare xv
magnesium treatment for myocardial infarction,
    conflicting results on 76
MAL meta-analysis 73
managed care
  in health care systems 11–12, 172
  influence on healthcare policy 218
  and insurance-based funding 180
  research-based evidence in 256–7
management
  evidence-based decision making in 9–12, 157–8
  quality of, and outcome of healthcare 12
management changes, and evidence based
    decision-making 54–57, 66
management decisions
  in health service management 9–10
  and resource allocation 172–4
management skills
  in healthcare 194–9
  of healthcare decision makers 2–3, 194–9
*Manual for Assessing Health Practices and Designing
    Practice Policies; the Explicit Approach* 242
MAP meta-analysis 74
marginal costs 136–7
maternal health, in Priority Research Programmes *227*
maternity service, assessment of quality of 141
media
  and clinical decision-making **202**, 206
  perception of health hazards by 188–9
medical directors, management skills of 3
medical education, effective methods of 216–17
medical literature
  on critical appraisal 241–2
  users' guides to 239–41

Medical Outcomes Study, and patient satisfaction 131
medically unexplained physical symptoms (MUPS) 14
MEDLINE (National Library of Medicine's
        bibliographic database) *8*, 62–3, 196, 230, *231*
    on effectiveness 115
    in the evidence centre 158
    on patient satisfaction 129
    on primary healthcare 168, 169
    on RCTs 80–1
    for reviews 72, 74, 221
    on screening programmes 49
    in search for therapy 30
    shortcomings of 76, 80–1, *223*
    on tests 42
meeting, need for evidence in 159
mega trials 79, 104
menorrhagia, and *Effective Health Care* bulletins 226
mental health, in Priority Research Programmes *227*
mental health services, evidence-based primary care in
        167–70
mental illness, and healthcare policy 55, 229
MeSH terms in searching for evidence
    on appropriateness 151
    on tests 42–3
meta-analysis
    of studies, search for 42–3
    in systematic reviews 73–4
    term from MEDLINE *231*
    on trials of outcome 107
methodology, quality of in RCTs 241
migraine, search for therapy for 30
mini-sabbaticals, in medical education 217
'more good than harm', concept of 18–20
'more good than harm' *see also* good:harm ratio
mortality rates
    as outcome measure 140, *141*, 142, 145
    risk-adjusted 143–4
    in studies of health service organisation 32–3
motivation
    in clinical practice 214
    in decision making 7
    in management skills 195
    in medical education 216–17
MUPS (medically unexplained physical symptoms) 14
myocardial infarction
    and antihypertensive agents 87–8
    and beta-blockers 107
    case-finding for 47
    effective management of 24, 79, 104, 141, *178*
        and purchasers' requirements 175, 176
    and magnesium treatment 76
    outcomes in hospital league tables 142
    and thrombolytic therapy, use of 22, 24, 83–4, *85*

'N of 1' trials 80
national differences, and healthcare policies 56, 187–8
National Health Service (UK) *see* NHS
National Library of Medicine (US), databases of 230, 234
National Research Register, of the NHS R&D
        Programme 233

natural experiments 71, 90, 145
necessity, in assessment of appropriateness 150–1
needs, evidence-based assessment of 5–6, 171–2, 229
neonatal intensive care, reviews of variations in 228
neonatal screening tests, introduction of 255
newsletters, of information for evidence-based primary
        care 169, *170*
NHS
    funding of, effects of on policy decisions 10
    reorganisation of, policy-making in 185–7
NHS Centre for Reviews and Dissemination (NHS CRD)
        224, 225–6
    publications of 225–6
    on search strategies 236
NHS Management Executive's (NHSME)
        District Health Authority Project 228–9
NHS R&D Programme
    and evolution of evidence-based healthcare xv
    features of research 69
    functions of 249
    National Research Register 233
    Priority Research Programmes 227
    and requirements for research-based knowledge 60–1
non-English language studies, in systematic reviews *75*
number needed to harm (NNH), in definition of
        safety 122
number needed to treat (NNT)
    and effectiveness of treatment 117
    and framing effect on results 85–6
    information on 232
    in safety, definition of 122
    in screening, appraisal of evidence on *51*
numerical tests, value of 37–8
NY Department of Health, and risk-adjusted operative
        mortality rates 143–4

objectives, in healthcare services 140–1, *187*
observational studies 70, 71
    on effectiveness 116, 117–19
odds ratio, in appraisal of evidence on effectiveness 117
oesophageal bleeding, clinical innovations in treatment
        of *165*
opinion-based decision-making 1
opportunistic implementation of evidence 255–6
opportunity costs 136–7, 139
oral contraceptives, and deep vein thrombosis,
        cohort studies on 123
organisation
    culture of, in decision-making 154, 183, 185–8
    development of, and use of this book xi–xii
    in evidence-based health service 155–6, 183, 185–8
osteoporosis
    doubtfulness of screening for *178*
    and *Effective Health Care* bulletins 226
outcome
    appraisal of 43, 71–2, 92, 197
    in decision tree 95
    of disease 103
    long-term, and observational research *70*
    and patient choice 207

and patient satisfaction 127
questions about 103–12
RCTs in assessment of 78, 79, *82*
searching for evidence on 145
of treatment 31, 90, 104
variations in 143–4, 145
outcome *see also* adverse effects; side-effects
outcome measures
in health service organisation 12, 18, 32–3, 135–6, 229
in healthcare policy *187*
of quality in healthcare 18, 102, 139–40, 142–4, *180*
outcome measures *see also* mortality rates
ovarian cancer, unproven value of screening for *23*, *176*, *178*
Oxford Regional Health Authority *see* Anglia & Oxford NHS Executive Regional Office
oxymoron, definition of 133

PACE programme 249, 253–4
Palmer, C.R., on analysis of disease clusters 189–90
patient
applicability of findings to the individual 110–11
perception of effectiveness of healthcare 114–15
patient *see also* elderly people
patient anxiety, and test results 39
patient care
assessment of 139–47
cohort studies on 90, 92
and healthcare policy 54–5
managed care systems 11–12
outcomes of 102
and patient choice 206, *207*
searching for evidence on 144–5
patient care *see also* outcome; process; quality
patient choice
in clinical decision-making 202, 203–12, 213
in trials 80
patient compliance, qualitative research on *99*
patient expectations
global rise in xiii
in healthcare 3–6, 18
consumerism 6, 18
and public education 172, 176
and satisfaction 126
patient leaflets, and patient choice 207, **208–9**
patient participation, and patient satisfaction 131
patient questionnaires, in qualitative research 100
patient responsibilities, in insurance-based funding 179
patient satisfaction
appraisal of evidence on 130–1
in appraisal of new treatments 163
dimensions of 126–9
and interpersonal relationships of care 115, 127, 128, 129, 131–2
searching for evidence on 129
patient selection
bias in 118–19, 123, 124
criteria in 105, 109, *110*
in effectiveness studies 118–19
and outcomes in hospital league tables 143

in patient satisfaction studies 130
in quality of care studies 145
and safety studies 123, 124
and study design *91*, 92
peer review, in research 69
pelvic pain, cognitive therapy in treatment of 14–15
peptic ulcer disease, clinical innovations in treatment of *165*
perceptual tests, value of 38–9
performance, appraisal of 195, 197, 214
personal costs, in decision tree 95
personnel, in evidence-based health service 155–7, 161, *162*
Pharmaceutical Benefits Advisory Committee (PBAC), guidelines of 163, **164**
pharmaceutical industry
and bias in results 84–5, 133–4
unpublished data of 61, 74
use of the media by 206
physical environment
and healthcare policy 13, 55
and patient satisfaction 127, 128
pituitary adenoma, and false-positive test results 39
placebo, in trials 104
policy making
evidence-based 183–92
in health service management 9–10
political factors
in decision-making 10, 28, 183, 185
in healthcare policy xiv, 54–5, 56
in implementation of research evidence 33
population ageing
global problem of xiii
and healthcare costs 4–5, 25, **26**, *26*, 201
power
inadequate, in trial results *223*
in RCTs 78, *79*, 81
rules *106*, *108*
to demonstrate adverse effects 123
predictive value, of tests 36–7
pressure sores, and *Effective Health Care* bulletins 226
preventive health programmes, economic evaluations in 137
preventive interventions, definition of 29
primary care management, of stroke, leaflet on **208–9**
primary research, evidence from 221
Priority Research Programmes, NHS R&D Programme 227
probability, in results 121, 147
process measures, of quality in healthcare 139–42
producer, of tests in healthcare provision 40
productivity, in healthcare 16, 17–18, 134–5
professional liberty, and decision-making 255–7
professional practice, and purchasers' requirements 175
professional skill
and patient choice on surgery 206, *207*
and perception of necessity 151
and quality of care 146–7
and risk in interventions 125, 143–4
professional standards, and patients' perception of effectiveness 114–15

professional training
    and appraisal skills 197–8
    and clinical innovations 176
    and evidence-based needs assessment 172
    and patient satisfaction 131–2
professionals
    comparison of treatment by 31–2, 71
    consultation with in GRiPP 250
    expectations of, in delivery of healthcare 5, 6–7
prognosis
    disclosure of and patient choice 211–12
    and predictive value of tests 36–42
project management, in implementation of evidence
        252–3
prospective studies 89, 123–4
prostate cancer, unproven value of screening for 23, 176
prostate surgery 42, 118–19, 229
prostatic hyperplasia, and *Effective Health Care*
        bulletins 226
provider, relationship with purchaser 16, 171–2
public concern
    and clinical decision-making **202**
    on disease clusters 189–90
public education, and patient expectations 172, 176
public health policies xiv, 55, 183, 188–92
    legislation in promotion of 191–2
publication of research 69, 221–33
    bias in, as barrier to good clinical practice *215*
    failures in 61–2
    registers of 232
    search difficulties 62–4
purchaser
    newsletter of evidence-based information for 242–3
    relationship with provider 16, 171–2
    and tests in healthcare provision 40–2
purchasing
    and cost control 112, 201
    decision-making in xiii-xiv, 9–10, 112, 157, 162–4,
        171–82
    and framing effect 85–6
    GRiPP in management of 178–9
    and health care needs assessment reviews 228–9
    and unproven interventions, reduction of 24

qualitative research 71, 99–101
quality
    assessment of 140–5
    of decision analysis 96, *98*
    of evidence 59–61, 68
    of healthcare 18–19, 113, 139–40, 145–7, 228
    and healthcare policy 54
    of management, and outcome of healthcare 12
    in practice, in screening 52, *53*
    in RCTs 81–2
    of research 19–20, 30–1, 69–101
    in screening programmes 49, 52
    of services, patient expectations for 6
Quality Adjusted Life Years (QALYs)
    and cost-effectiveness 136
    as outcome measure 112, *146*

questions
    on applicability of research findings 83, 109, *110*
    for appraisal of review articles *74–5*
    on outcomes 103–12
    in studies on patient satisfaction *130*

raised blood pressure, and stroke prevention **208–9**
RAND Health Sciences Program 150–1
randomised controlled trials (RCTs) 78–80
    in *ACP Journal Club* 232
    appraisal of 81–3, 83–4
    on effectiveness 116
    in experimental research 71
    on healthcare policy 32, 55
    methodology of 78, 81, 82, 225
    promotion of by purchasers 177
    on public health interventions 188, 190
    representation of 84–6
    on safety 123
    on screening 49
    searching strategies for 80–1, 237
    terms from MEDLINE *231*
    on test performance 43
    on therapy 31
    unsuitable subjects for *70*
reference management systems 196, 198–9, 247–8
Register of Cost-Effectiveness Studies 232
registers of published research 232
registers of research in progress, unpublished evidence
        233–4
relative benefit, in evidence on effectiveness 117
relative risk 117, 122
relative risk reduction, and framing effect on results 85–6
relevance of evidence 109–10, 113
    on appropriateness 152
    on cost-effectiveness 138–9
    on effectiveness 119, 125
    and patient choice 110–111, 204, 207
    on patient satisfaction 130–1
    on policy making 187–8
    on quality of care 145–7
    on safety 125
relevance gap, in requirements for research-based
        knowledge 60
renal disease, healthcare needs assessment 229
representation, of RCTs 84–6
reproduceability, of findings on services *110*
research 8–9, 69–72
    application of in GRiPP 178–9
    appraisal of quality of 30–3, 69–101
    design 30, 43, *44*, *231*
    economic evaluations in 137
    on effectiveness 116–18
    funding, and bias 133–4
    implementation of 33, 44, 249–57
        in health policy and management changes 57
        in screening 52
        in tests 44
    and index of interest 59–61
    methods 197, 225

for evidence on effectiveness 116
  in evidence-based journals 232
  in studies of health service organisation 32
  on outcome 104–8
  poor quality, as barrier to good clinical practice *215*
  searching for 30–3
  unpublished 61, 74, 233–4
research-based knowledge, and effectiveness in the
  NHS 182–3
resources
  and clinical decision-making 13–15, 172–4, **202**
  constraints on xviii, 33, 219
  in decision-making 1, 3, 7, *8*, 10
  in evidence-based needs assessment 171–2
respiratory disorders, resources for 174, 229
results, of systematic reviews *75*
retrieving, evidence *see also* searching 198–9
retrospective studies 89
reviews *see also* systematic reviews 197, 221–2, *223*
rheumatoid arthritis, clinical innovations in treatment
  of *165*
risk
  absolute risk, in definition of safety 122
  absolute risk reduction 85, 232
  and applicability of research findings to the
    individual 111
  level of, and quality of management 12
  reduction of, and public health policies 190
  in safety, definition of 121–2
risk factor analysis, in evaluation of public health
  interventions 188–90
risk-adjusted operative mortality rates 143–4

Sackett, D.L. et al, *Evidence-Based Medicine:
  How to Practice and Teach EBM* xvii, 235
safety 121–2
  appraisal of and searching for evidence on 122–4, 125
  evidence for, in audit 159
  and healthcare policy xiv
  in new treatments, appraisal of 163
  and quality, evidence on *144*
  of therapy, assessment of 31
scanning, in searching skills 65, 196
schizophrenia, reviews of variations in 228
screening programmes 29, 46–53
  in decision analysis of 95–6, **97**
  as public health interventions 188
  tests in 23–4, 34
searching for evidence 59–66, 198–9, 235–7
  on appropriateness 151
  by purchasers *242*
  on case-control studies 88–9
  on cohort studies 91
  on decision analysis 96
  in decision-making 2–3, 161
  on effectiveness 115, 138
  on healthcare policy making 55–6, 187
  as management skill 157, 195–6
  and patient choice 204
  on patient satisfaction 129

on qualitative research 101
  on quality standards 144–5
  in RCTs 80–1
  on safety 122–3
  in systematic reviews 74
  on tests 42–3
  on therapy 30
seat belt legislation, controversy regarding 191
secondary research 72
sellers, pharmaceutical industry as 133–4
sensitivity
  and effectiveness of screening 46, 47
  MeSH headings for 43
  of tests 35–40
sensitivity analysis, in decision analysis 96, *98*
services, observational research on 71
severity of illness, and outcome 140, 143
side-effects of interventions
  assessment of 31, 147–8
  in decision analysis 95–6, *98*
  and patient choice 207, 211–12
side-effects of interventions *see also* adverse effects
sign, definition of 34
size, of trials, and confidence intervals 107–8
smoking, qualitative research on *99*
social environment, and health 13, 55
social status, in illness 14
somatoform disorders 14–15
South and West Regional R&D Programme 227
specialist services, access to, reviews of variations in 228
specificity, of tests 35–40, 46
staffing policy, cohort studies on 90
standard texts, on critical appraisal 241–2
standards, of care 140, 141–2
'stopping starting', of unproven interventions 23–4, 44,
  176, 254–6
stroke
  healthcare needs assessment 229
  management of *178*, **208–9**
  preventive interventions 117
  in Priority Research Programmes *227*
  rehabilitation and *Effective Health Care* bulletins 226
study design, in cohort studies 91, 92
study protocol, in research programme 69
subcutaneous continuous infusion pumps, and patient
  preference 80
subfertility, and *Effective Health Care* bulletins 226
subgroup analysis, appraisal of 82, *83*
subject specialist bibliographic databases 230–2
surprise threshold, in analysis of disease clusters 189
surveys 93–4, 123
symptom, definition of 34
systematic reviews
  in *ACP Journal Club* 232
  appraisal of 74–7
  dimensions of 72–4
  on effectiveness 116
  in experimental research 71
  MEDLINE search strategy for 236
  need for evaluation of 3
  preparation of 225

on public health interventions 188
on safety 123
on screening 49
searching for 74, 221–4, 236
on tests 43
on therapy 31
of trials, computer access to 59
uses and abuses of 77, 169
systematic reviews *see also* CDSR

taxation, in health service funding 179–81
technology
    impact of xiii, 5–6, 7, 25–7, 165–6
    in Priority Research Programmes *227*
telephone access, to information for evidence-based
        primary care 168, 169
tests
    appraisal of 43–4, *44*, *45*
    decision-making about 34–45
    definition of 34–42
    diagnostic, and increased volume of treatment 41–2
tests *see also* screening
textbooks
    in the evidence centre 158
    shortcomings of 22, *215*, *223*
thalidomide, failure of appraisal of evidence in 23
therapy
    decision-making about 29–33, 162–4
    definition of 29
therapy *see also* treatment
thiazide, relative risk of impotence from 122
thrombolytic therapy, in myocardial infarction
        management 22, 24, 83–4, *85*
time, lack of, as barrier to good clinical practice *215*
toxic waste, and politics 28
training
    in appraisal skills 197–8
    for evidence-based decision-making 161, *162*
    programmes, in CASP 243–5
    in reference management systems 199
    in searching for evidence by managers 196
treatment
    after diagnostic tests 41–2
    after screening 47, 50, *51*
    effects of, studies on 87, 90
    unnecessary, and false-positive test results 39
treatment *see also* adverse effects; outcome;
        side-effects; therapy

trials *see* clinical trials; research
tuberculosis control, economic appraisal of 139
TURP (transurethral resection of the prostate gland),
        bias in studies of effectiveness 118–19

UK Online Users Group (UKOLUG) 247
UKOLUG newsletter 247
unintentional injuries to children, and *Effective Health
        Care* bulletins 226
unpublished evidence 61–2, 74, *75*, 77, 233–4
use of evidence, training for evidence-based
        decision-making 161
Users' Guides to the Medical Literature 239–41
utilisation, of services, and appropriateness 149–50, 151
utilities, in decision analysis 95, 96, *98*

validity, of evidence *74*, *82*
values, in healthcare decision-making 1
variability, in perceptual tests 38–9
varicose vein treatments, healthcare needs assessment
        229
venous thrombosis, outcome of 102
ventricular fibrillation, observational research on
        treatment of *70*
virus diseases of the central nervous system, research
        interest in 59–60

Web *see* World Wide Web
Wessex Regional Health Authority, Development
        and Education Committee 227
Wide Area Network, and information for
        evidence-based primary care 168
World Wide Web
    in the evidence centre 158
    Evidence-Based Healthcare Toolbox xvii
    on evidence-based primary care 169
    in resources for decision makers *8*
    on search strategies 235, 236, 237
    sources of reviews on 227

York Database of Abstracts of Reviews of Effectiveness
        see Database of Abstracts of Reviews of
        Effectiveness
York University *see* NHS Centre for Reviews and
        Dissemination (NHS CRD)